FIBROMYALGIA RECOVERY

FIBROMYALGIA RECOVERY

FIBROMYALGIA SECRETS REVEALED

**FIBROMYALGIA TREATMENT PROGRAM
STEP-BY-STEP GUIDE**

ISKRA HARLE
Holistic Medicine

iUniverse LLC
Bloomington

FIBROMYALGIA RECOVERY

Copyright © 2010, 2013 by Iskra Harle, Holistic Medicine.

All rights reserved. No part of this book may be used or reproduced by any means, graphic, electronic, or mechanical, including photocopying, recording, taping or by any information storage retrieval system without the written permission of the publisher except in the case of brief quotations embodied in critical articles and reviews.

iUniverse books may be ordered through booksellers or by contacting:

iUniverse LLC
1663 Liberty Drive
Bloomington, IN 47403
www.iuniverse.com
1-800-Authors (1-800-288-4677)

Because of the dynamic nature of the Internet, any web addresses or links contained in this book may have changed since publication and may no longer be valid. The views expressed in this work are solely those of the author and do not necessarily reflect the views of the publisher, and the publisher hereby disclaims any responsibility for them.

Any people depicted in stock imagery provided by Thinkstock are models, and such images are being used for illustrative purposes only.
Certain stock imagery © Thinkstock.

ISBN: 978-1-4502-4453-4 (sc)
ISBN: 978-1-4502-4454-1 (ebk)

Printed in the United States of America

iUniverse rev. date: 07/11/2013

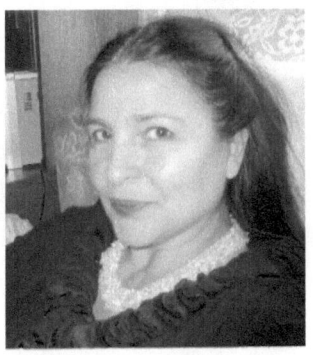

My efforts to understand fibromyalgia have been richly rewarded. The results are beyond my expectations. Fibromyalgia is a multifactorial condition, very serious and therefore must be addressed in all its different aspects.

This publication has only one aim, to give you a succinct and perspicuous Guidance of how to recover from Fibromyalgia.

Part 1—'Fibromyalgia secrets revealed' is about the individual features, the chain of biochemical reactions within the body and environmental factors that cause fibromyalgia.

Part 2—'Fibromyalgia Recovery Program' is a detailed protocol with a step-by-step Guide to fibromyalgia reverse.

Iskra Harle
Health Practitioner Holistic Medicine
Member of The Royal Society of Medicine
www.healthonline2000.com

The world is not the same without you
In loving memory of my dad

DISCLAIMER

Every effort has been made to make this document as complete and accurate as possible.

However, there may be mistakes in typography or content.

The information given here is designed to help you make an informed decision about your health. It is not intended as a substitute for any treatment that may have been prescribed by your doctor.

If you suspect that you have a medical problem, we urge you to seek competent medical help.

Therefore, this document should be used as a guide only.

The author and publisher do not warrant that the information contained in this report is fully complete and shall not be responsible for any errors or omissions.

The author and publisher shall have neither liability nor responsibility to any person or entity with respect to any loss or damage caused or alleged to be caused directly or indirectly by this publication.

INTRODUCTION

A personal experience

Fibromyalgia had always been on my doorstep; back pain, moody periods, mild depression, insomnia . . . But 8 years ago it pounced on me. In such a short time! In 3 months I was disabled.

Instead of reconciling myself to all of this I found my own way to recovery.

I cured myself! I conquered Fibromyalgia!

It is a great feeling.

Sometimes I had my dreads—maybe my fibromyalgia symptoms could return. But as time went by there was no recurring sign of Fibromyalgia Syndrome. I am still free of pain, free of stiffness, free of causeless tears, free of depression, free of all Fibromyalgia symptoms. And not only this, in addition, my general health has improved.

I am absolutely confident that my Protocol can help everyone to recover from Fibromyalgia and all concomitant conditions; back pain, depression, fatigue, hypothyroidism etc. You just need to follow the Fibromyalgia Recovery Protocol. I believe this is the best protocol for fibromyalgia, as it covers all aspects of the condition—from the root causes through 1-2-3 guidance and on to complete recovery. Do exactly what I did and you will be Fibromyalgia free.

When years ago I was diagnosed with Fibromyalgia Syndrome I heard only discouraging opinions. Nobody believed a cure was possible. Everyone said, 'It's for life, nothing really helps, and it's going to get worse'. I ignored all this. I said to myself: 'I am not going to be disabled for life! I am going to find a fibromyalgia treatment and to recover from Fibromyalgia!'

I had a pretty good life. I wanted it back—and, I got it!

What future had I with Fibromyalgia? A life with pain killers and antidepressants? Increasing the doses . . . and where is the limit? If you look around, you will find that what the market has to offer for fibromyalgia is mainly painkillers and anti-depressants; which only alleviate the symptoms. This is not a real cure for fibromyalgia.

This wasn't for me.

I don't want a substitute for real health! Real health is life without pain killers, with no antidepressants, with no medicine! So, I needed to search in a different way. Taking into account that official medicine still struggles with fibromyalgia diagnosis and treatment, I had no choice but to look for an alternative method—natural, harmless and by all means, **to cure Fibromyalgia**.

I remembered the legend about Hygeia and her sister Panacea, (the two daughters of the Greek God of health, Asclepius). They both had the gift of healing, but they were helping people in very different ways. Panacea used powders, mixtures, tablets. She was constantly looking for some magic tablet that would cure all illnesses. On the other hand, Hygeia taught people the Art of Life, taught them **WHAT A HEALTHY STYLE OF LIFE IS**, taught them to follow

THE LAWS OF NATURE, and that *this* is the way to **achieve** and keep **good** physical and mental health.

So, I followed Hygeia's way—no medicine, all natural fibromyalgia treatment.

I did my fibromyalgia research. I read about fibromyalgia symptoms, about fibromyalgia pressure points and trigger points, causes of fibromyalgia. I read the comments of support groups about different fibromyalgia treatments . . . and all this information confirmed my conviction that there is no medication for fibromyalgia that really works, even some medications act as a trigger for the symptoms.

Gradually I developed an alternative fibromyalgia treatment, a recovery program that works. I cured myself.

During these years I realized how many people suffer from fibromyalgia and were going through the same agony like me. They need help And I CAN help!!!

I wrote down my recovery program, my fibromyalgia diet, my recipes, my exercises.

So, here we are. I am going to take you with me on the same journey of recovery, through the same fibromyalgia diet, nutritional supplements for fibromyalgia and other healthy tips that helped me. I am absolutely sure they are going to help you as they have already helped me, but-not-only-me.

I should admit, I could not keep my findings only to myself and had already started helping people using the same recovery program.

I am receiving emails like this:

"I have suffered FM for over 5 years and from once being a very active person, I find it very difficult to accept this disability. My achy muscles and stiff joints are more confined to my ankles, knees, elbows and wrists as well as fingers. I do yoga once a week, so I feel this helps my back considerably. However my main concerns are my "tension headaches" which can be unbearable!! I don't think my sore head has gone away in years!! It's always there although it just feels some days are better (or worse) than other days. My concentration is terrible, which means that during my working day I am lucky to get 30% of what I am really capable of doing. My energy levels are not good either and can require naps through the day, although they don't necessary make me feel any better. Walking the dog can be a struggle at times when I am bad. Please can you help?"—John, UK

"I am 25 years old and I've been suffering from muscle stiffness, joint aches and pains, insomnia, tension headaches, upset digestive system which results in a bloated stomach, constipation, poor concentration, it's always foggy in my head, really bad mood swings, irritability, anger (all the time), flu like symptoms for the last four years. I have to stay in bed for about 9 to 10 hours to feel that I've had enough sleep/rest. Also just walking for a few hours makes me really exhausted and when I get some time I have to take a nap. I have fallen arches and due to this I was told by the foot specialist that it is the reason why I get stiff muscles and it will go away (this was four years ago)! I have seen specialists who have taken rheumatoid arthritis tests, and they have come back negative. I was put on Amitriptyline to treat neuropathic pain but this didn't help, so I stopped taking that medication.

I did ask the rheumatoid specialist if it was fibromyalgia and she said she didn't know, so now I don't really know what to do about my health other than its making me very depressed and its affecting me physically and emotionally. Hopefully there is something that can be done." Janet, Portsmouth

People of different ages, mostly women, share their pain and anxiety, and are asking for help. I feel immense satisfaction when **after a single week, they feel the difference**: 'I feel great.' 'My head is not foggy anymore!' 'I haven't felt like this for ages'. The doubts are gone and they stick to the Program.

This fibromyalgia treatment recovers not only your **physical body sufferings**, but your **mental status** as well. You don't only feel how the **pain and stiffness goes away**, but you have more energy, you are alert, your bloating is eliminated, soon you begin to **feel happier**, your **sadness and tears**, your **depression and despair disappear**.

This treatment works so well! But if you expect some kind of unusual method, some magic, something extraordinary? I have to say, there is nothing unusual in this treatment. Nothing unusual at-all!!! **Everything you need is in your local food shop/supermarket and health store**—just common, but appointed foods—the best diet for fibromyalgia.

If you have any doubts, please, feel free to share with your doctor, I am sure, you will be given the 'OK' for this fibromyalgia treatment as it was given to everyone that has already asked.

Every time you shop you are probably passing these products on the shelves. You might even have some of them at home.

The combination of them and **the way of preparation** is what works so magically for your recovery from Fibromyalgia. **You are going to be surprised at how quickly it works, how easy it is to follow the protocol.** It is amazing how these simple, well known, ingredients really work from the very first day. You will be surprised, when you realize that you not only can, but you also would like to stick to the fibromyalgia diet. **This is not a medical treatment.** This is a **style of life that suits your body** and stands against fibromyalgia. This is a style of life that you will feel comfortable with. You are going to like it!

The protocol

This Treatment protocol is original as an idea and unique with its simplicity and effectiveness. The treatment consists of complete detox of the body and at the same time introducing the right nutrients for the cells.

The improvement begins from day one. This is **The Fibromyalgia Treatment that can cure you.**

If you can follow an EASY Step-by-Step Guide with full explanations of your daily routines, **you will succeed** and you will never look back.

The recovery program layout provides you with:

Detailed daily regimen, Step by Step Guide for the next 8 weeks and **further.**

The recovery program is **suitable for both women and men.**

This is a step by step guide for your complete recovery. The protocol acquaints you with the foods that are suitable for your body. They improve the body biochemistry and put it back into balance.

There are also specific exercises. I call this 'Lazy Gym'. It is really as easy as it sounds.

Another good feature of the fibromyalgia diet is that there are **no unusual foods** and probably you have most of the products at home. If not, your local shop will provide you with what you need. **There are NO complicated preparations**, and everybody—man or woman, even teenagers can do it. It is **less expensive** than usual food costs and takes **very little time for preparation**.

In fact, there is nothing difficult in the treatment.

Due to the structure of the protocol, every day is marked with improvement.

Here are the daily feedbacks from a very busy young student—Janet from Portsmouth. Before starting the treatment she asked me if the treatment is going to affect her study, her exams. She was thrilled by the fact that her memory improved thanks to the treatment. Her daily feedbacks are very similar to everyone else, due to the structure of the Fibromyalgia protocol.

Day 1—I didn't have the usual sick feeling. I also noticed that I didn't feel bloated like I usually do.

Day 2—Again I didn't feel bloated or nausea, which was nice. Still had some muscle tension and a slight tension headache but I didn't take any pain killers . . . Just forgot to mention I didn't have any lower abdominal cramps today.

Day 3—Well today, surprisingly, I didn't get up with a tension headache! It was really nice to have a **clear head**. My muscle aches and pains were less than normal and my sore throat was not as bad as it usually is. I didn't feel bloated, my constipation and cramps have gone.

Day 5—I felt more awake and had **more energy** than usual.

Day 8—I feel like my digestive system is cleaner, the muscles in my neck are not as tense as they used to be.

Day 10—I didn't feel aches, pains or stiffness at all, other than stiffness in my hands and feet. I've also found that my skin feels really soft especially on my face, which is what I told you earlier on the phone. I feel very **alert** at the same time.

Day 12—I felt very **alert** this morning. I just found it took less time than yesterday to settledown and study. I felt that my head was much clearer when it came to studying. The only muscle stiffness I felt was in the hands and feet. I have had **a lot of energy** today. It's nice to feel awake and alert and not have a fuzzy head, I also felt a little **happy too :-))**

Day 13—I still feel alert and not as tired as I usually do, my brain has actually been working!! **Ha—ha! I didn't have any other stiffness as usual and I'm finding it easier to stretch, it's not as painful as it used to be, it's more fun and relaxing.**

Day 14—I have to admit since I started the treatment it's got much better; and I'm finding that I'm getting better at waking up and concentrating on usual routines much better. **It's definitely improved since!!**

Day 20—I don't feel as irritable as I used to be.

Day 26—I also keep **getting up an hour before my alarm** goes off.

Day 32—I find that eating regimen throughout the day has helped me **concentrate and focus properly**.

Day 35—I didn't have any muscle aches and pains.

Day 36—I am very alert and cheerful and my muscle aches and pain had gone.'

I wish quick recovery to everyone!

Iskra Harle

Part 1
FIBROMYALGIA SECRETS REVEALED

INTRODUCTION

Fibromyalgia is a chronic disorder of the skeletal muscles. The ailment manifests itself by stiffness and pain in the muscles, extreme fatigue and depression.

Fibromyalgia could appear at any age. Ninety per cent (90%) of those who suffer from Fibromyalgia are women. Fibromyalgia is not a typical male illness, but ten per cent of Fibromyalgia sufferers are male. This is largely due to today's car-and-computer-lifestyle. In 1993 Israeli doctors reported their observation that an unexpectedly high number of children met the criteria for Fibromyalgia. Since then specialists pay more attention to children's pain. Where one lives also plays a part, as it is in the Northern climes such as the Scandinavian countries (like Sweden and Finland), Canada, US etc, that Fibromyalgia most often occurs. According to the official records, 2% of the population of the UK and US suffer from Fibromyalgia. There are grounds to reckon the real figure is significantly higher.

For years, Fibromyalgia was not recognised as a real medical condition. Fibromyalgia has been linked incorrectly to rheumatic diseases, to depression or denoting it as psychosomatic. Because of the specifics of the disease, patients have often been directed to arthritis specialists. Although there is pain in the area of the joints, Fibromyalgia is not a form of arthritis. It does not cause inflammation, nor does it damage the joints, muscles or other tissues in the body as arthritis does. Some of the symptoms of Fibromyalgia tally with symptoms of other illnesses like chronic fatigue syndrome, depression etc.

There are a large number of people with all the symptoms, but with no diagnosis. Nowadays, medical institutions carry on researching Fibromyalgia, but scientists still have no conclusion about a chain of causation or remedy that works for Fibromyalgia. The mystery of the illness comes from the fact that there are no definitive medical markers to confirm Fibromyalgia. The traditional check up, blood tests and X-rays, show a healthy person and the sufferers are often turned away. A typical report from Fibromyalgia sufferers sounds like this:

Email: 'I have not been diagnosed with Fibromyalgia yet. However, I have all the symptoms. I have been working with several doctors and they have not been able to find out what is wrong with me. They have even begun to "brush me off," once seeing me every other week, now only wanting to see me once a month, some not even returning my calls.' A. B.

Patients are the ones who are best informed on the specifics of their condition and share helpful information between each other. As the medics have not established a test to confirm Fibromyalgia, there is no proper medical cure offered for this disease. Despite all of this, **there is a treatment protocol that reverses Fibromyalgia.**

The curative method was established after in-deep research into the fine biochemical processes in the human body. The idea of the root cause of Fibromyalgia presented itself clearly, and has been tried and tested successfully since then. A process of experiments ensued, with close observations on the results. Finally a treatment was discovered that leads to the complete reverse of Fibromyalgia. In addition, the method is natural and harmless.

Some patients have been consulting their doctor about this treatment. The opinion of all of the medical practitioners has been: 'I don't know whether it is going to help you or not, but it definitely will not harm you.' Our first thought when we are not well is to look for medicine. This treatment is different. It involves no medicine whatsoever and below you will find all the answers you need about **Fibromyalgia and how to cure it.**

SYMPTOMS

The first indications of Fibromyalgia may come during early childhood. Children sleep restlessly and have difficulty getting out of bed in the morning. There could be a flu-like illness with a variety of throat problems, like sore throat, tonsillitis or even thyroid and adrenal gland disorders. There may be lung problems, coughing or sinusitis and a running nose. Often persistent 'cold hands and feet' have been noticed. Kidney disorders occur. Memory could be affected, which gives frustration at school age. Proneness to tears or mood swings could be one of the early signs of Fibromyalgia.

HERE ARE THE MOST OFTEN REPORTED SYMPTOMS OF FIBROMYALGIA:

- Chronic pain and stiffness in the soft tissues in the body (muscles, tendons and ligaments) around the neck, shoulders, waistband, hips, spine, elbow, knee, legs and face. These areas are stiff, numb, tingly and swollen. Morning stiffness is a very typical symptom.

- Difficulty in sleeping (insomnia). There is a pain at night that disturbs rest and in time becomes unbearable.
- Lack of energy or extreme fatigue. There is tiredness and unwillingness to get out of bed in the morning.
- Depression, anxiety, dizziness, poor memory, poor concentration. This indicates the involvement of the central nervous system in most cases. Some sufferers report that they are plunged into blank despair and driven to consider suicide.
- Fungal infections, Irritable Bowel Syndrome (IBS).
- Sensitivity to chemicals (preservatives in food, drugs etc.). Liver enzyme irregularities create chemical sensitivities.
- Parallel with the increasing typical Fibromyalgia symptoms (muscle pain and stiffness), is observed sensitivity to: intense light, low temperature, windy weather, draughts, loud sounds and noise, odours and pollen. There are sinus pains, headaches, skin problems, constant infections; Red blood cells sticking together; Sexual hormone problems, including menstruation irregularities.
- Fibromyalgia has been diagnosed in 20% of those suffering from Lupus erythematosus. Fibromyalgia often develops after polio, miscarriage, hypothyroidism, parathyroid glands disorders, heartburn, mouth ulcers, swollen lymph nodes, rib cage pain.

The illnesses that accompany Fibromyalgia appear in different organs and systems in the body: kidneys, liver, lungs, intestines, nervous system, endocrine system, sexual system etc. Organs so different in their structure, shape and use appear to have something in common—their functions slow down, parallel with the manifestations of Fibromyalgia. There is a reason for it as outlined below.

THE CAUSES OF FIBROMYALGIA

There are a number of suppositions and theories about the cause of Fibromyalgia and all of them circumnavigate the truth; this includes the theory of an injury or trauma that affects the central nervous system, the theory of metabolic disorders that decrease blood flow, or the theory of an infectious agent. In 2007 Dr. John C. Lowe, from Fibromyalgia Research Foundation, announced the theory of thyroid hormone deficiency. According to his study 54% to 68% of fibromyalgia is due to thyroid gland disorder.

I would say all of them are looking in the right direction, but there is a lot more.

Vitamin D deficiency consequences

In context of fibromyalgia, vitamin D deficiency is found to affect the body in two ways. It is essential for 1) **maintenance of the capillaries** and 2) causes **Homeostatic disorder**.

The word vitamin comes from Vita, which in Latin means Life. Vitamins enable essential bodily functions to be performed effectively. Vitamin deficiency causes a number of serious health issues. The body is able to synthesize some vitamins by itself, while others have to be supplied by food. One vitamin is so important for the body's functions that nature has provided two ways of supplying it and also, possibility to store it. First of all, the body is able to synthesize it. If this source is unavailable, there is a second way in which the body can receive it through food. This is vitamin D.

What is vitamin D? It is a peculiar steroid compound, fat-soluble vitamin. The body is able to store it for a long time and retrieve it on request, when needed. Vitamin D comes in many forms—D1 (Lamisterol); D2 (Ergocalciferol)—it is synthesised by plants; D3 (Holecalciferol) is synthesized in the human skin; D4 (Dihydrotachisterol), etc. Thirty-seven forms of vitamin D have been identified.

Different forms of Vitamins D have different origins but very similar structures and properties. Their biological influence over the human body has also been found to be very similar. Vitamin D3 (Holecalciferol) is produced in the human skin when it is exposed to ultra-violet light with a wave length of 290-320 nm which is part of natural sunlight. Vitamin D3 is available in large amounts in fish oil and especially in cod liver oil. Fish (herring, mackerel, tuna, turbot, etc.) and all sea food contain vitamin D3. Vitamin D is also found in eggs, butter, bio yoghurt, cream, feta cheese, cheese, and dark green leafy vegetables. The best source of vitamin D remains the one produced in the skin, under the influence of sunlight. For northern regions, where sunlight is insufficient, obviously the best source of vitamin D is fish, caviar and sea products; and they should be included every day in the diet.

Neither a deficiency, nor an over-dose of vitamin D is of benefit to the body. The skin has a fine regulative mechanism for the synthesis of Vitamin D under the influence of sunlight. When the skin becomes darker, the production of vitamin D slows down. Synthesis starts again when the skin becomes lighter. As is so often the case, nature finds her own balance. Health problems usually come when we disrupt that balance through our lifestyle.

Vitamin D is multifunctional. The presence of vitamin D in the body prevents muscle weakness and pain. It is essential for the nervous system and for healthy bones. It is prescribed for rickets, for osteomalacia (softening of the bones), osteoporosis, caries (tooth decay), lupus vulgaris (skin tuberculosis), psoriasis, larynx and kidney tuberculosis, scrofula, hypoparathyroidism, ear and eye problems, etc.

Sara Hiom, head of Health information at Cancer research UK, says: "There is evidence to suggest that vitamin D plays a role in keeping the cells healthy". Practically, there is no part of the body that does not need vitamin D.

From vitamin D deficiency starts the chain of factors that causes Fibromyalgia. I would say vitamin D is the most important of them all.

How does its deficiency affect the body? What is the connection between vitamin D and Fibromyalgia? What else besides vitamin D leads to Fibromyalgia? Would it be enough to take vitamin D supplements? Why doesn't everyone suffer with Fibromyalgia?

Vitamin D conversion and Fibromyalgia

When contained in food, vitamin D is broken down and assimilated in the **small intestine** in the presence of gall bladder juice (bile). There is a requirement though—the food has to contain some amount of fat for vitamin D to be assimilated. Actually most of the natural sources of vitamin D contain fat—fish, eggs, feta cheese, etc. In the blood, attached to the proteins, vitamin D is transported into the **liver** where it undergoes a transformation to another, more active form—25-hydroxiholecalcipherol or **calcidiol**. This new compound is five times more potent than its precursors. The transformation continues into the **kidney**, where the final substance—1-alfa, 25-dehydroxiholecalcipherol or calcitriol, obtains ten times more potency than its precursors. This final substance is the one that the body needs—**calcitriol**.

Vitamin D3, produced in the skin, goes through the same process of transformation in the liver and kidneys.

The intestines, liver and kidneys are the three main parts in the process of vitamin D conversion. Malfunction of any of them affects vitamin D conversion to calcitriol. For example: there are clinical evidences that many patients with a well functioning liver, with a sufficient level of calcidiol, still have calcium metabolism disorders. The weakest link in this case is their kidneys.

Calcitriol, the active form of vitamin D, takes part in **calcium** metabolism. The calcium comes from the food, through the intestines, into the blood. Calcium, contained in the blood (1% of all Ca in the body) is essential for many biochemical reactions, including contraction of the muscles. (See below "Calcium")

What is the connection between vitamin D and Fibromyalgia?

The active form of vitamin D, calcitriol, possesses hormonal properties. This compound influences a genetic apparatus of the small intestine cells to produce a specific protein, which is essential for absorption and transportation of calcium. When vitamin D is insufficient, there is a low level of calcium in the blood. Calcium is then not absorbed from the food. The blood has to be supplied with calcium. Parathyroid glands regulate calcium in the blood and bones, so, **parathyroid glands** being involved in the process. They raise a secretion of parathyroid hormone. Then starts mobilisation of calcium from the bone tissues (the bones contain 99% of the body's calcium) and also suppression re-absorption of the phosphates in the kidney. In a healthy person, calcium and phosphate react in opposite ways. As the blood calcium level rises, the phosphate level falls. While the kidneys decrease phosphates in the blood, the bones render calcium into it. At the same time, the activity of alkaline phosphatase sharply increases. The body's regulative mechanisms (buffers) are activated to maintain **homeostasis**, to reinstate chemical balance. But this process is not always successful. That is the bottom line for the chronic illnesses, including Fibromyalgia.

Homeostasis

Homeostasis is a property of the body that maintains its internal dynamic equilibrium. It is a ceaseless process of regulating the internal balance of different parameters—pH (alkalinity—acid balance), temperature, blood glucose; the kidney remove excess of water, salt and urea from the blood—the main waste products; the lungs—carbon dioxide, etc. In this process are involved most of the organs in the body, including the liver, kidneys, skin, endocrine system—parathyroid glands, thyroid gland, hypothalamus etc. What follows when one or more of the organs work inefficiently? It is then that we observe a Homeostatic disorder. There are different scenarios depending on the organs involved, but they all lead to one result, the body accumulates **metabolic waste products (toxins) and the pH index becomes acid.**

A healthy liver would deal with the toxins for a while, until it became obstructed or its cells are damaged from the toxins. The kidneys would release the water soluble waste products for a while, until they became exhausted and damaged. The kidneys are often a weak point for fibromyalgia sufferers along with other organs, rich in capillaries.

The tissues, naturally abundant with blood capillaries, are most affected from the excess of metabolic waste products. According to Gray's anatomy, an abundance of capillaries are found in the part of the intestines that assimilate nutrients, the kidneys, the thyroid and parathyroid glands, the brain. In addition, the capillaries in these organs are the smallest in the body, easily congested and damaged and as a result, the organs become sluggish.

The muscles are also abundant with blood capillaries (compare the red colour of the muscles with the white colour of the cartilage (where are presented only lymph vessels). The muscles perform two actions—contraction and relaxation. **How do the muscles react to an excess of metabolic toxins? With a contraction, with a painful, long lasting contraction; the first sign of Fibromyalgia.**

The lack of vitamin D unlocks a chain of biochemical reactions and leads to acid-alkali imbalance and accumulation of calcium and phosphorus in the blood and soft tissues, including the muscles. All this starts with a vitamin D deficiency.

Homeostatic disorder is the real reason for Fibromyalgia.

Homeostatic disorder is not a disease. It is a misbalance within the body. In this case it is auto-toxication due to the inability of the body's buffer systems to deal with metabolic waste products.

I would like to emphasize this: **MEDICINE TO RESTORE HOMEOSTASIS DOESN'T EXIST**. Maintaining the homeostasis is a natural process which requires no medicine, but knowledge of the natural processes within the body and applying it in your daily life in order to achieve an optimum condition of the tissues in the body in order to recover the function of organs involved in the homeostasis maintenance. The necessary steps to achieve it are set up in Fibromyalgia Recovery Program (read below).

The blood toxins affect all the muscles in the body, not only skeletal, but also cardiac and smooth muscles. Contraction of the **skeletal muscles** causes stiffness and pain; and these are the most frequently reported Fibromyalgia symptoms. (See below "Skeletal Muscles").

The **cardiac muscle** also endures contraction. As a result of this, the heart's animation force is reduced. Low blood pressure occurs, which affects all organs in the body, manifested by lethargy, tiredness, fatigue, and specific response from other organs. All hollow internal organs (intestines, stomach, kidneys, bladder, spleen, veins and arteries, etc.) are built from **smooth muscles**. Their contraction slows down digestion, causing constipation, the need to frequently pass water, depression, etc. Homeostatic misbalance causes neurological and muscle complications. Sufferers complain of bone pain, chest pain, head ache, decreased visual and mental activity. The entire body suffers the consequences of the toxication.

FM does not cause physical damage, nor inflammation or wounds, but pain, tiredness and depression. Here it must be noted that the traditional physical **examination** occasionally reveals signs of disease, but is otherwise normal. (For more on diagnosis see below at "FM examination")

Homeostasis and buffering systems

Homeostasis is a **fine balance** between content, reactions and other characteristics of the blood and other liquids, as well as a number of physiological functions. The **pH** is a concentration of hydrogen ions in the blood. The pH in the body's liquids vary—from 4.5 (acid) in prostate cells to 8.5 (alkali) in bone cells. An acid-alkali balance in the blood requires the proportion between carbonic acid and bicarbonates (alkali reserves) to be 1:20. Then the pH remains constant.

Buffering systems

During daily activities and due to illness, alterations to the pH occur all the time. Buffering systems function within the body to neutralize the excess of acid or alkali products. Usually there is an excess of acid products. The buffering systems are highly effective, and any changes to pH are restored quickly to the normal indexes. For example, there is very little difference in the pH count of the arterial and venous blood in a healthy person: 7.35 and 7.33, but they are kept constant. A **buffer** is a substance that resists changes in pH level. Blood buffering systems have different kinds of buffers—phosphates, bicarbonates, haemoglobin, and proteins. The buffering capacity of the blood depends on the volume of the buffers. Additional regulating factors are respiratory (breathing) and kidney mechanisms. The organs involved in keeping acid-alkali balance are also the liver and the skin with its sweat glands.

Food

Knowing what foods to add to your diet and what to avoid can make a big difference in your health. The food you eat every day is a powerful acid-alkali regulatory mechanism. Unsuitable food, poor digestion and insufficient assimilation of the nutrients, affect homeostasis.

Unsuitable are acid forming foods, like meat, sugar, alcohol.

Digestive system disorders, very often Candida infections, cause malnutrition—a lack of proteins for cell renovation, a lack of enzymes, which are proteins, a lack of minerals and vitamins, including vitamin D.

Inappropriate food causes homeostatic imbalance, usually acidosis. When the body's own buffering systems fail to maintain the homeostasis, the only alternative is appropriate food.

Vitamin D and capillaries

Every cell, tissue and organ in the body needs specific nutriment to exist, for cell-division, to recover itself, to fulfil its function, etc. For the capillaries, the essential substance is vitamin D. **Vitamin D is the most important nutrient for healthy capillaries.** Lack of vitamin D affects the condition of the capillaries. In the body new capillaries are formed all the time, while others become stunted. Capillaries are present all over the body. Practically, every single cell is in contact with a capillary, where the metabolic processes in the cells are performed. The arterial part of the capillaries supplies the cells with nutrition. Through the venous part are evacuated the metabolic waste products. The capillaries are also a depot for the blood. Blood vessels are supplied with very sensitive cells—sensors that react quickly to changes in the blood **homeostasis** (see above). **Muscles and organs in the body like the kidneys, thyroid glands, parathyroid glands, ovaries, etc. are very rich in capillaries. They are the ones that suffer most from vitamin D deficiency** and consequently homeostatic changes.

Vitamin D insufficiency from childhood reflects on the quality of the capillary net. A child, growing up in an environment that does not provide enough vitamin D (indoor lifestyle, climate features, etc.) develops an inferior capillary net and organs function, which affects the person's health during their whole life. Fortunately, the process is reversible. Any positive changes immediately stimulate new capillary growth.

Inferior musculoskeletal capillaries

Functionally the more active the organs are, the larger the capillary net is, which corresponds to their need for a large blood supply. The capillaries are the smallest blood vessels. Their network is that part of the body where metabolic processes are fulfilled. The smallest capillaries are found in the brain (which in some conditions can cause depression in FM sufferers) and mucous membrane of the intestines (hindering assimilation of nutrition). The largest capillaries are found in the skin (the organ of detoxification) and the bone marrow. The static (red) skeletal muscles are very rich in capillaries. FM recovery program announced below increases the blood flow through the muscles.

Capillary inferiority is one of the main reasons for FM. **The poor functional condition of the capillaries, like spasms,**

high permeability, rupture etc., does not contribute to a proper nutritional supply for the muscles and metabolic toxin elimination. Tendency to thrombosis and high cholesterol levels slow up the blood flow and impede metabolism. When capillary spasms occur (due to acidosis, stress), the immediate reaction is stiffness and/or pain in the muscles. This is a most frequent trigger for the typical FM symptoms. The contraction and relaxation of the arterioles determine and regulate the blood flow through the capillaries. To implement contraction and relaxation, the body needs the availability of specific substances—microelements, vitamins, etc. Calcium ions take part in the conduction of contractions. The body has a huge reserve of calcium ions: 99% of the body's calcium is located in the bones. While the body's needs to conduct a contraction are well satisfied, it is quite opposite when it comes to implement a relaxation. The nutrients are supposed to come from the food. Eating the right food will supply the nutrients that provide muscle relaxation. This is not only vitamin D. Vitamin D supports the condition of the capillaries, so that nutrients can enrich the cells.

How to open the capillaries appears to be an object of profound research. Recently scientists have studied the connection between so called Substance P and FM. Substance P is associated with pain, mood disorders, anxiety, stress, respiratory rhythm, etc. There is a theory, that Substance P is the main chemical responsible for sending pain signals from the body to the brain. Capsaicin is a compound which is present in the capsicum vegetable (chili peppers). The precise mechanism of action of capsaicin is not fully understood. It is believed that it relieves pain by reducing Substance P. Whatever the truth is, the Iskra Health System practice shows that after two hours of burning sensation, Capsaicin relaxes the contracted and painful muscles. The effect continues for about 3 days.

According to recent scientific research, Substance P is also a vasodilator, which increases blood flow through the capillaries and therefore the metabolic processes, by widening the blood vessels and by releasing nitric oxide from the endothelium.

Endothelium is an epithelial tissue. It covers the inner surface of the blood vessels and also composes the blood and lymph capillaries. Therefore the well being of the skeletal muscles depends also on the condition of the epithelial tissue.

There is a special feature. During the initial process of recovery, following principals of the Iskra Health System, for about two weeks your usual pain level will increase slightly. You have to be prepared for this as it is part of the healing process. It takes time (2 to 6 months) for the existing capillaries to open, new capillaries to grow and to enrich the cells, metabolic waste products to be reduced, and the body to get into balance.

Calcium

Calcium ions present in the blood are involved in muscle contraction, transmission of nervous impulses along nerves, and blood clotting. They contribute to the cell's structure and many enzyme reactions. Our bones and teeth hold a huge storage of calcium. They contain about 99% of all calcium in the body. The remaining 1% is in the blood, tissue fluids and the soft tissues. A small amount also exists in the liver.

Calcium metabolism is affected from: lack of vitamin D, mucous membrane inability to assimilate it from the food, liver and kidney inefficiency and parathyroid disorder. The Ca shortage affects further biochemical processes. The body is starved of Ca, and needs to take some from the bones. Parathyroid glands send a message to the bones to release calcium. As the whole body's functions are already disturbed, this process is also imprecise and could be observed either hyperparathyroidism or hypoparathyroidism. An excess of calcium enters the blood. Excretion, mainly through the kidneys, is impaired. The result is hypercalcemia. It is the other extreme: an excess of calcium is being deposited in the joints, blood vessels and soft tissues which causes additional pain. Hypoparathyroidism causes 'pins and needles', spasms. It affects all the muscles, including those in the hands and feet, and face as well.

MORE REASONS FOR FIBROMYALGIA

Tissues and organs involved in FM condition

Assessment

When the body runs out of vitamin D, Fibromyalgia symptoms occur. Vitamin D deficiency and its conversions obstructions are the main factors, causing FM but there is more. Below is presented the analysis on tissues and organs, according to their inherent (from birth) and acquired (from unsuitable lifestyle) conditions in relation to fibromyalgia. Some of them are naturally strong and resistible, while others are weak and easily susceptible to the adverse effects of their environment.

Here are the results of an assessment of randomly chosen FM sufferers, all of them with an advanced form of FM. Patients' own observations, combined with a detailed medical questionnaire, were essential for this assessment.

We are going to look at the following groups of organs and tissues as indexes:

1. Cardiac (heart) and smooth muscles
2. Stomach
3. **Lungs, intestines and connective tissue** (ligaments, tendons, membranes).
4. **Kidneys** and attached **adrenalin glands; areas of the throat (thyroid gland, parathyroid glands)** and **blood vessels**—capillaries, veins, arteries. Special attention must be paid to the **capillaries**. The static skeletal muscles are very rich in capillaries.
5. **Skeletal muscles**. These are permanent tissues but are dependent on the condition of their supportive tissues—connective tissue and capillaries.
6. Liver—the main organ of detoxification.
7. Bone system, including cartilage.
8. Nervous system.
9. Endocrine system.
10. Sexual system.

Patient/Index	P1	P2	P3	P4	P5	P6	P7	P8	P9	P10
1	NAD	X	X	X	X	X	NAD	X	NAD	X
2	NAD	NAD	X	X	X	X	X	X	NAD	X
3	X	X	X	X	X	X	X	X	EF	X
4	X	X	X	X	X	X	X	X	X	X
5	X	X	EF	X	X	EF	X	X	X	X
6	X	NAD	X	X	X	X	X	EF	X	X
7	X	X	X	X	X	X	NAD	X	X	X
8	NAD	X	X	NAD	NAD	NAD	X	X	NAD	X
9	NAD	NAD	X	X	X	X	NAD	X	NAD	NAD
10	X	X	X	NAD	NAD	X	X	X	X	X

P—Patient; X—weak tissue or organ; EF—external factor; NAD—no abnormality detected

Observation:

1. All of these patients have shown an insufficient function of the **capillaries** and **connective tissues**. (The skeletal muscles, and especially the static ones, are very rich in capillaries. The connective tissue sheets wrap round the muscle and the ligaments, connecting the muscles to the bones and lamellae). Kidneys, adrenalin glands; thyroid and parathyroid glands; lungs and intestines are from the same groups and do not meet the requirements for the body's homeostasis. The role of the kidneys was explained above. The rest of the organs are also involved in homeostatic processes.
2. The second position for insufficient function is held by the tissue of the skeletal muscles. It has to be stressed that two of the cases have shown naturally strong muscles, but at the same time the lifestyles of P3 and P6 lacks of physical activity, and therefore muscular metabolism is considerably low.
3. Next is the bone system: including cartilage and the bone marrow (part of the immune system). Nine out of ten FM sufferers have by the nature a weak bone system, which explains why FM sufferers have been directed to rheumatologists.
4. The liver is well known as the chemical laboratory of the body. It neutralises toxins and takes part in vitamin D metabolism. Patient N6 has naturally a strong liver, but alcohol abuse (an External Factor) has damaged it, so the chain of synthesizing the active form of vitamin D—calcitriol, is broken.
5. Patient N9 has a naturally strong digestive system, but has a Candida infection (an External Factor) which affects calcium absorption.

6. This is followed by the sexual system. The connection between the sexual system and the muscles consists in the influence of sexual hormones on the muscles.
7. The functional strength of the heart and the stomach share the penultimate position. Cardio-vascular insufficiency takes part in FM symptoms—tiredness, fatigue. Inferior stomach function has an effect on protein digestion and therefore muscle repair.
8. The strongest position is held by the nervous tissue and glands. They belong to the group of permanent, firm tissues. The nervous cells are very sensitive to any lack of oxygen. FM is a chronic condition, so there is not a lack, but a shortage of oxygen. This causes dizziness, poor memory and depression.

Conclusions:

Fibromyalgia occurs when there are inferiority of capillaries, connective tissue and kidneys from birth. In most cases, skeletal muscles are a weak point and it is those that are affected by FM. The additional weak tissues contribute to the wide variety of FM symptoms. Lack of movement burdens the existing chronic ischemia of the capillaries, which results in a disturbed nutrient supplier, and slows up the action of the buffering systems and the elimination of the metabolic waste products from the muscles. Muscle fibres and connective tissues respond by painful contraction.

The removal of the Fibromyalgia syndrome requires:

- **Vitamin D sufficiency,**
- **Improvement in the functions of the organs, and especially the liver and kidneys,**

- **Acceptance of eating habits and nutritional products that support acid-alkali balance** (and do not produce excess of metabolic waste products which are difficult to eliminate), and
- **Adoption of a lifestyle which provides physical activity, appropriate eating habits and regular detoxification** (involving all the detox systems in the body).

To remain healthy, we need to bear in mind the individual features of our body.

The organs in the body have to be considered as interconnected vessels. If one of the organs is weak, this affects the others. Capillaries and connective tissue are present all over the body. Insufficient function of the capillaries and connective tissue affects the whole body, but mostly the organs that contain high amounts of them. In accordance to their needs, some organs are created with more capillaries than others. In first instance capillary insufficiency affects the skeletal muscles but also the endocrine glands in the throat area, kidneys, lungs, intestines and brain. General health deteriorates as gradually more organs depart from their inherent work. The low blood circulation affects the muscles in different ways, but in this case also creates difficulties to maintain the homeostasis.

The first element is a poor nutritional supplier. Hypoxia appears (oxygen shortage). The blood usually contains enough glucose and amino acids, but they are not metabolised because of a shortage of oxygen. As a result there is scant nutrition in the muscles, and consequently a lack of energy and fatigue.

The second negative element is a hindrance in the elimination of metabolic waste products, for the same reason—the capillary condition. All this affects homeostasis. Waste products build up—in the muscle tissue, mainly lactic acid; in the area of the joints, calcium crystals; which irritate nerve endings and provoke the well known stiffness and aching. The connective tissue sheets that cover muscle fibres and ligaments at the ends shrink and shorten. The muscles are hard to the touch, and painful when stretched (FM symptoms).

Another impediment comes from a build-up of lipid plagues, which lessen the vessel's lumen. Reduced haemoglobin and other substances thicken the blood. All this contributes to a difficult detoxification.

Exercise and sports activity improves blood flow. A sedentary style of life turns the initial FM symptoms to chronic.

Mucous membrane and Fungal infections

The **mucous membrane** of the small intestines is the place, where the nutritional substances from the food enter the blood. To perform properly, the mucous membrane should be in healthy condition. Anything that disturbs its function affects nutritional absorption. Inflammation of the mucous membrane of the small intestines (enteritis), Irritable bowel syndrome and fungal infection are very often at the root of the problem. A bloated stomach and cramps in the abdominal area are a signs for IBS and food allergies. Fungal infection is a very common reason for a lack of calcium in the blood and following homeostatic disorder. A white coated tongue signals a fungal infection. To recover the mucous membrane functions is one of the first tasks of the required treatment.

For most FM sufferers, the trigger is a **fungal infection**. Candida Albicanis causes more than 85% of the cases. It is known as thrush or yeast of the digestive system. It is a normal inhabitant of the human body. Candida Albicanis is found in the mouth of 30-60% of healthy people ('Clinical evidence'—BMJ Publishing group). Fungi develop best in an acid environment—pH 3-6.0 (Common microbiology—S. Vlahov, A.Ivanov). A strong immune system and appropriate food are able to suppress its development. Candida infection occurs when the protective system is genetically weak or becomes weak, and/or the food consumed on daily basic is unsuitable. Conveyance occurs between infected people or on fomites. Transition of fungi from the infector over and over again is the most frequent way for the spreading of a Candida infection and its persistence. The fungi develops in the mouth (white coating on the tongue is visible) and intestines. It harms the body in different ways. Fungal infection affects digestion and the absorption ability of intestines as well as the elimination of waste products through them. Candida is seen in the white coating that compactly covers the mucous membrane and prevents absorption of specific nutrition from the affected area. It causes inflammation of the mucous membrane underneath, disturbing the secretion of the digestive glands and immune system cells, located therein (80% of the immune system is located in the digestive system), as well as the poor condition of the capillaries. Candida contaminates the blood with its own toxic products, mycotoxins, which the blood transports to all cells in the body, which increases the overall toxic condition. The nutritional balance is infringed. For example potassium ions play a role in muscle relaxation, storing glycogen in the muscles (for energy) etc. A deficiency causes prolonged and painful muscle contraction and fatigue. The body's reserves of potassium are limited (only 0.32% of all the minerals in the body). They are supposed to be regularly replenished. Potassium comes from food, so the appropriate products have to be consumed, but the digestive system also has to be able to assimilate it.

Cardiovascular system features +

The cardiovascular system includes the heart, the arteries, the capillaries and the veins. Here we can add the lymph vessels also.

<u>Heart</u>

Cardiovascular insufficiency and **low blood pressure** are also preconditions for FM. The heart is working ceaselessly, yet it never tires. The cardiac muscle fibers are a permanent tissue. As FM does not damage tissues and organs, there are no observations of cardiac disease. At the same time as the persistence of metabolic acidosis and increasing level of metabolic waste products, the blood pressure gradually falls and with time, this becomes a permanent condition. Low blood pressure explains the tiredness and fatigue that FM sufferers experience. This is a part of the overall picture of FM. The cardiac muscle could be genetically strong or weak. But this doesn't change the 'behavior' of the heart in FM patients. Lowering blood pressure is a protective reaction of the body's self preservation mechanisms. An additional reaction is the narrowing of the blood vessels. The body is trying to prevent the existing excess of toxins in the blood from entering the cells. This action is performed by the usual reaction of the muscles in such a situation—contraction. All the muscles in the body are affected. This causes stiffness and pain in the skeletal muscles. The function of the internal organs slows down and the body becomes lethargic.

What do we do to get rid of this pain and stiffness? Usually we would take pain killers, but this is only a temporary measure. Gradually we have to take increasingly stronger pain killers, and eventually we become dependent on them. We could get pills to dilate/enlarge the blood vessels but there is no point in this as it would be against the body's own self-preservation reactions. The right way to relieve this condition is to evacuate the toxins and recover the homeostasis. Then the pain will disappear, the capillaries will automatically open; the blood pressure will increase to the normal level, and your strength will return.

Often we hear a widespread opinion: 'High blood pressure is dangerous. It is better to have low blood pressure.' The truth is that only normal blood pressure is good for you. Low blood pressure (LBP) also has serious negative consequences for the human body. LBP causes chronic hypoxia (organs lack oxygen). There is observed cyanosis (blue-reddish color of the tissues and organs) due to the increased level of reduced hemoglobin. The third main consequence of LBP is swelling; as a result of stagnant kidneys. LBP affects the entire body. The main damage is due to the chronic hypoxia:

1) micro-hemorrhages as a result of laceration (tearing) of the capillaries;
2) Dystrophy and atrophy of parenchyma;
3) Tissue's components being destroyed (as a result of a lack of oxygen) and replaced by connective tissue;
4) Fibrosis—the tissues and organs become dense. The hypoxia also causes chronic fatigue and depression.

The assumption that a lack of sleep (because of night pain) is causing the fatigue has its place, but this is not the main reason for it.

Lymph vessels

While the capillaries in the skeletal muscles are abundant, the lymph vessels are present only in the connective tissue around the muscles—in tendons and in the sheaths. The lymph flows in one direction only—from the periphery of the body to the center, and carries minute globules of fat, some proteins, lymphocytes, etc. In comparison, the blood carries mainly water-soluble substances, while the lymph carries mostly fat-soluble substances.

The blood is pumped by the heart contractions, but the lymph liquid moves thanks to the muscle movement.

It has been discovered that the lymph vessels are more numerous in epithelial tissue—skin and mucous membrane, the two areas where Vitamin D enters the body. As with blood, the lymph liquid is able to coagulate.

Sedentary style of life

Who suffers from Fibromyalgia? Why doesn't everybody suffer from FM?—Natural predisposition is the main reason, but your style of life influences whether FM will develop or not. FM is a condition of the skeletal muscles. The parts of the body which are less active are those which suffer. Lack of movement sets the pattern for muscle pain and stiffness.

Sedentary style of life, lack or absence of movement in the skeletal muscles is one of the main preconditions of FM.

A sedentary style of life triggers FM. We are frequently having too much TV-time or computer browsing. Students under strenuous study can be affected, cashiers, book-keepers etc. FM can be developed after being bedridden following an injury or trauma etc. Our life increasingly depends on the car. To save time we drive instead of consciously finding an opportunity to have a walk. By car we bring our children to school and bring them back home; by car we go to work. We even drive to the local shops.

The muscles need movement. This movement brings life into the muscles. The deficiency of movement that precedes FM does not predispose a good oxygen supply. Without oxygen there is no strength in the muscles, there is tiredness and fatigue. The regeneration of the muscles depends on movement. Only connective tissue is able to multiply in an anaerobic environment. Movement contributes to proper nutritional supply and also—that is how the muscles get detox.

Muscles

There are 3 main kinds of muscles in the body—skeletal (static and dynamic), smooth and cardiac muscles. There is an essential difference in their way of detoxification. The smooth and cardiac muscles are involuntary. They are regulated by inner factors. Their movement and vibrations never stop. For skeletal muscles it is different. They are voluntary muscles and without our will and effort they will not move.

Lack of movement results in: the peripheral blood circulation slows down, metabolic processes slow down; the nutrients are exhausted and the voluntary muscles heap up metabolic toxins. Excess of toxins affects particularly static muscles. More or less dynamic muscles are involved in the daily movements—to stand up or sit down, to walk the distance between the house and the car, for short run etc. Dynamic muscles are designed to do short time movements. Static muscles have different characteristics and without special effort involving the will, it is difficult to provide detoxification.

Skeletal muscles

Skeletal muscles are those affected by their own capillary insufficiency, the condition called FM. Striped fibers are the specialized tissue of skeletal muscles. The common tissues in skeletal muscles that serve the muscle fibers are: connective tissue, blood vessels and nerve tissue. The connective tissue forms sheaths that cover the bundles of muscular fibers (perimysium) and tendons that attach the muscles to the bones, cartilages, ligaments, skin or to other muscles. The blood vessels are: arteries, they supply with nutrition; capillaries where is fulfilled the exchange of nutrients and metabolic waste products; veins evacuate the metabolic toxins. There is a profuse amount of nerves. Larger arteries and veins are found only in the perimysium. The striped and especially the static striped muscles are abundant in capillaries and anastomosing branches. Lymph vessels are present only in the tendons and in the connective tissue sheaths of the muscles. The skeletal muscles are highly specialized to provide one of the most important vital functions—the voluntary movement and posture of the human body.

Static and dynamic skeleton muscles

There are two kinds of skeletal muscles—dynamic DM (white) and static SM (red). FM affects especially the **static skeleton muscles (SM)** that relate to the body's posture.

Locations of the static muscles

The static muscles are mainly multi-jointed. Such muscles are paravertebral muscles (spine area), upper limb flexors, m. trapezius—descending fibers (shoulders and upper back), m. quadrates lumborum (lower back, flank), ischiocrural muscles (hips-thigh), m. gastrocnemius, m. soleus, m. rectus femoris, m. iliopsoas, m. pectoralis major, m. levator scapulae.

Special features

Here are some special features about static (SM) and dynamic (DM) muscles. They have a number of differentiations.

- Static muscles are red in color. They have more capillaries than dynamic ones. Dynamic muscles are called white due to the less number of capillaries.
- SM are mainly multi-jointed, DM are one-piece.
- SM are under the extra-pyramid nerve regulation. DM are under pyramid nerve regulation.
- SM contractions change slowly and this contraction is tonic i.e. increases vitality. DM contraction changes quickly and it is tetanic, they harden when active.
- SM get tired slowly, DM get tired quickly.
- Glycolic enzyme activity in SM is aerobic, so they need more oxygen than DM (anaerobic). Glycolic enzyme activity in SM is low but they have a high level of lipid metabolism. Metabolic waste products are water and carbon dioxide, which is easy to eliminate. For comparison, DM metabolic waste product is mainly lactic acid, which is the reason behind the pain after dynamic physical activity of an untrained person. Lactic acid is the intermediate product of the anaerobic break down of carbohydrates. DM have low lipid metabolism.
- When the muscles heap up glycogen and proteins, a considerable amount of potassium is engaged in the

cells. Insufficiency of potassium ions leads to salient muscle tiredness and the muscles are unable to heap up glycogen which is used for energy. This concerns mainly DM. For SM the lipids are the main energy source. In the condition of aerobic metabolism they dissolve fats. From a biochemistry point of view, the cardiac muscle is similar to SM, it is also aerobic, and needs a lot of oxygen.
- Myoglobin (protein that stores oxygen in muscles) content is higher in SM.
- In certain pathological conditions SM and DM react differently. SM decrease their ability of stretching, their tonus increases and their ends draw near to each other. Prolonged muscle contraction occurs, which is very painful (FM syndrome).
- SM get tired slowly, DM—quickly.

The best short distance runners have 90% dynamic muscles and 10 % static, while marathon runners have 92% static and 8% dynamic muscles. The proportion between static and dynamic muscles is determined by genetic factors. Nothing can change this proportion. There is no evidence that under training this proportion yields any change. The muscles have an obvious unity of function and structure. The dynamic muscles do fast movements but for a short time (sprinters). The static muscles (which provide posture) get contracted slowly and get tired slowly, as is the case with Marathon runners ('Remedial massage manual'—T.Kraev, L.Todorov). Probably women have more static muscles than men. Women are able to do static, low mobility work for a long time, while for men this is not as easy. Obviously it is not about the patience, we believe the woman possessed more, but it depends on the predominance of the kinds of muscles. This is one of the reasons more women to suffer from FM than men—90% as opposed to 10%.

FIBROMYALGIA EXAMINATION

Acidosis and muscles reflex reactions

There is a reflex reaction of the muscles induced by different organs of the body—central nervous system, internal organs, etc. Unhealthy diet or a motionless professional posture, high toxic level lead to specific reactions from the muscles, mainly in their tonus—contraction of the SM (pain, stiffness) and weakness of the DM (tiredness).

Muscles reflex reactions manifestations:

1. Increase of muscles fiber tonus (spasm). If you pass your fingers across muscles fibers, you will feel they are stretched as rope. This is a most common reaction and it is very painful.
2. Myalgia—if you touch or press specific points on the body, it is painful. The pain can also be spontaneous; with or without muscle spasm.
3. Deep zones of high sensitivity to pain (hyperalgesia)
4. Congealed and stiff muscles which remain after a spasm is gone.
5. Muscle hypotrophy—weakness, lifelessness, flabbiness; a muscle reduces its volume.

The symptoms of metabolic acidosis are specific and the diagnosis can be difficult. Arterial blood gas sampling is essential to confirm metabolic acidosis. The sample has to be taken from an artery, which is more uncomfortable and difficult than vein-puncture. Arterial blood test is not a common practice, as there are also a number of risks such as gangrene of a finger or loss of the hand functions from spasm or clotting.

Satisfying FM diagnosis could be made by the American College of Rheumatology diagnostic procedure. Diagnostic consists of examination of 18 points on the body. If 11 of them are sensitive to pressure, the FM condition is considered to be a fact. In addition to those 18 points I consider the points on the spine as well (as shown in the drawing below).

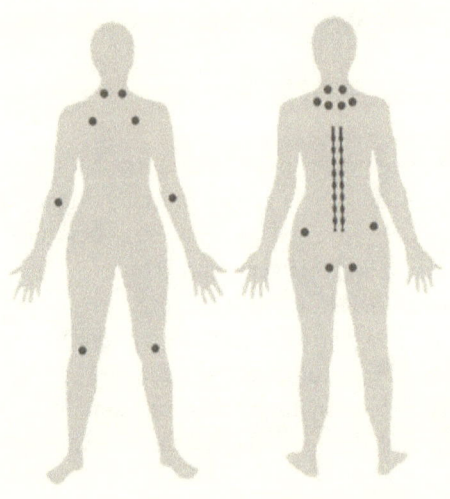

Part 2
FIBROMYALGIA RECOVERY PROGRAM

The diet that cures Fibromyalgia

INTRODUCTION

Fibromyalgia is a **Homeostatic disorder** which leads to muscle aches, stiffness of ligaments and tendons, fatigue, depression etc.

To recover from Fibromyalgia you need to **focus on two main tasks:**

Task One: **Total body detoxification,** which supports

Task Two: **Rehabilitation of those tissues and organs involved in maintaining Homeostasis.**

The treatment described below is oriented to **cure the disease**, not only to alleviate the symptoms.

Following the treatment program as directed, you will make life changes you'd never thought possible.

Here we are going to concentrate only on the process of your recovery.

The treatment uses natural remedies—expedient foods, herbs, juices, mild exercises; **all natural products** with no harmful side effects.

Because of chemical sensitivities established in FM, medicine is not recommended.

The Recovery Program is a schedule of specially chosen ways for detoxification, nutrition and exercises. It consists of two parts—**DAILY ROUTINES** and **GUIDANCE**.

The **Daily Routines** part enumerates the ingredients: how much to take (doses), when to take them, how long to take them.

The ingredients are multifunctional and only the right combination of them, as directed in the program, works.

The section entitled **Guidance** comes next. There you will find, in detail, exactly what you are to do. The Guidance section is an integral part of the Recovery Program.

You will need to concentrate on your health for about two months. This time is sufficient for you to get to use all the new healthy tips and changes. After this . . . just keep going.

After two months most of you will have no FM symptoms and may decide you are fine and do not need to follow this healthy lifestyle. **But *please*, *please*, do not cut off your treatment yet!** The organs involved in Homeostasis maintenance **need time for full recovery**.

> **-The recovery process continues long after the symptoms have disappeared-**

Human biochemistry—The chemistry of the human body has a complex character. Countless biochemical reactions are conducted all the time. But, there is a specific feature. Each of these reactions needs exact substances, in certain amounts. If even only one of them is missing, the reaction cannot be conducted. As a result your health gradually goes down.

Nutritional supply—To regain our health we need to give the body those nutrients it needs. How to supply the body with the missing nutrients? There is only one way—by eating the food that contains them, by eating the right food. Obviously it is not what we have eaten during the past years. We need to make changes in accordance to the nature and features of our body.

Toxins—What happens with the excess of unused substances? They become waste products (toxins) which clog the vessels and organs. They change the biochemistry in the body and provoke corresponding reactions, like headaches, dizziness, tiredness, stiffness of the muscles etc.

These toxins have to be eliminated from the body. The common way of detoxification works only towards water dissolved toxins. Reality shows us that there are more kinds of toxins that need to be dissolved and evacuated from the body. Only then will the body regain its balance, i.e. Homeostasis.

A new lifestyle—

The 1ˢᵗ task of this Recovery Program is towards **Total Detoxification**.

The 2ⁿᵈ task is—**Nutritional Supply**.

There is a 3ʳᵈ point I want to stress.

You need to keep your body in chemical balance. How? Turn this Recovery Program into a **Style of Life**, as I did.

During the following 2 months you will get used to this healthy lifestyle. You will find that you are not going to miss any food you like. The changes are only towards the doses. **The results you are going to achieve are worth this little effort.**

Good Health is not a goal, it's a journey.

NUTRITION YOUR BODY NEEDS

Have you ever thought how many basic Nutritional Substances your body needs?

Some of these substances we use unconsciously—like air and light. They are not on the shop shelves and we often take them for granted.

We discover the insufficiency of these substances only when our body is not able to **absorb** enough of them. For instance smoking and pulmonary diseases impede the body's metabolism and its use of air (oxygen absorption and expulsion of carbon dioxide and other toxic gases).

There are 4 basic types of nutritional substances: **LIGHT, AIR, WATER** and **TRADITIONAL FOODS** (of vegetable and animal origin). The deficiency, excess, or misbalance of any of these brings a chain reaction: disturbance of the regular functions of the organs, resulting in disease. At the start of this process the body resists, but not for long.

Without **air** the body can live a few minutes; without **water** several weeks; without **food** several months.

The substance of **light**; especially ultra-violet light, is a special category and nature has foreseen 2 ways to satisfy the body's needs for it. The lack of natural light can be compensated indirectly by specific kinds of foods, but only if the body is capable of absorbing them.

In addition to the 4 kinds of nutritional substances, we should add one more category; **MOTION**. Movement and exercise are essential for the muscle tissues in the body.

The main part of my FM research was to identify the insufficient nutrients and especially those substances the human body cannot synthesize. I had to account the common denominators in the style of life and eating habits of FM sufferers.

TOXIC SUBSTANCES—A KEY FACTOR

This presentation is not designed to convince you that tobacco, alcohol and the toxic environment are harmful to your health. We all know this, and you will make your own decision on these.

Also, some medications have side effects. They affect the functions of the liver, kidney and digestive organs. Check your medicine's side effects and consult your doctor for replacement, or possibility to pause them.

Bear in mind, **the condition of the liver, kidney and digestive organs is a key factor for recovery from Fibromyalgia.**

TRIGGERS TO FIBROMYALGIA

The main factors that trigger Fibromyalgia are the following:

- metabolic toxic products (internal factors),
- fungal infections—Candida/Thrush (external factors)
- and the side effects of medication.

HEALTH FROM THE INSIDE

The Recovery Program presented below includes elements that will purge the body daily of:

1. water-soluble and fat-soluble metabolic toxins,
2. calcium deposits around the joints and in the endocrine system,
3. stones in the kidney and the liver,
4. excess mucus and fungal growth, which make the absorption of the useful nutrients difficult.

> ONLY BY PURIFYING THE INSIDE
> OF THE BODY IT IS POSSIBLE TO
> ACHIEVE REHABILITATION, TO
> CURE FIBROMYALGIA, AND TO STAY
> HEALTHY.

RECOVERY PROGRAM OBJECTIVES

The objectives of the Recovery Program are as follows:

1. Improvement of nutritional assimilation
2. Improvement of nutritional synthesis

3. Detoxification
4. Introduction to—Insufficient Nutritional Substances-
5. Giving enough time for complete recovery
6. Building up a healthy lifestyle as a preventative measure against the recurrence of Fibromyalgia.

HEALTHY EATING TIPS

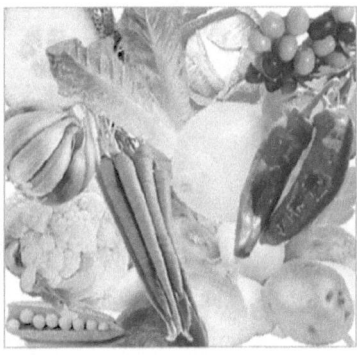

1. In the morning eat **bran**: to clean the digestive system and ease the assimilation of food during the day—wheat bran, oat bran or if you have intolerance to wheat products (celiac disease), use rice bran. All of them available in the health shops.

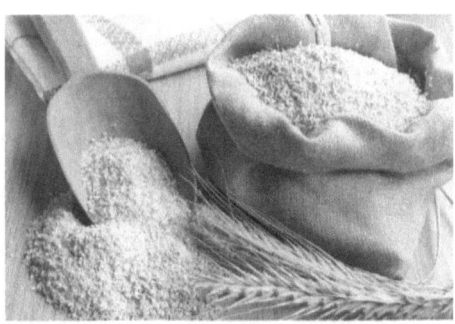

2. Eat all foods **fresh and raw** where possible. Cook only products which you cannot eat raw (potatoes, rice, beans, lentils and other pulses); fish and meat should be baked.
3. NO LIMIT to the quantity of **RAW food**. Eat as much as you like.
4. **RAW SALAD** at lunch and evening is your main food; this is what your body really needs.
5. **Salad dressings**. Healthy options:
    – Oil + vinegar; Use sunflower oil, sesame oil etc. + Red wine vinegar, white wine vinegar or apple vinegar (make sure they have no added chemicals, such as synthetic acetic acid, tartaric acid. **Do not use malt vinegar**).
    – Oil + lemon juice (freshly squeezed).
    – Tomato sauce from fully ripe tomatoes. Use a blender.
    – Life/bio yoghurt is a tasty dressing for lettuce salad.
6. There is a **LIMIT to COOKED** food.
    It can be no more than **20%** of the meal.
    e.g.: Weigh your lunch. If it is
    1kilogram (2.2 pounds) it has to consist of
    800grams (1.8 pounds) raw food +
    200grams (0.4 pounds) cooked food)
7. Have a large salad (80% of the meal) for **lunch** + 20% carbohydrates (energy).
8. In the **evening** eat a large salad (80% of the meal) with fish (20% of the meal). Any fresh or frozen fish is suitable, but make sure it contains no

preservatives. You can also use plain tinned fish (For example: Tinned Tuna fish is now available in fresh water (avoid brine = salt).
9. Use wholegrain rice (brown or white). Do not use polished rice. The most valuable nutrition of rice is in the bran.
10. The best way for the body to get fatty nutrients is from raw sources such as nuts, sunflower seeds, sesame seeds, olives, cold pressed oils and unsalted butter. These fats should not be heated during food preparation. Add no salt.
11. Substitutes for refined sugar are sweet fruits and honey.
12. If you are **allergic** to some of the recommended foods, start the treatment without them. To prevent allergens entering the body the intestinal membrane produces a lot of mucous, building a barrier to the allergen, but also stopping the absorption of useful nutrition.

    First you need to **eliminate the allergy**. So, take plenty of raw carrot juice 3-5 times a day for 2 to 8 weeks. This should be enough. Then add to your diet the products you've been allergic to. The allergy should be gone. Then continue as prescribed.
13. **NO SALT, NO PRODUCTS THAT CONTAIN SALT.**
14. Do not add salt to your meal.
15. **NO COFFEE, COLA DRINKS, TEA,** no **FOODS THAT CONTAIN PRESERVATIVES**
16. **NO SWEETS** or biscuits, chocolates, etc.
17. **NO MILK**—Milk is a food only for young mammals. They only have the enzyme (lactase) necessary for its proper digestion.
18. Avoid processed foods.

LET'S START KEEP RECORDS

Before starting on your recovery, take time to
LIST ALL OF YOUR SYMPTOMS (p48).
Date this and sign it.

This is important so that you link your progress with the program. Otherwise as soon as you feel better you may give chance the credit, fall back to your old habits, get sick again and, (strangely enough) say that the program didn't work!

Keep a daily record of:

a) your progress,
b) your relapses,
c) **your deflections from the Program.** *Learn from your mistakes.*
d) **Keep a record of your blood pressure weekly.**

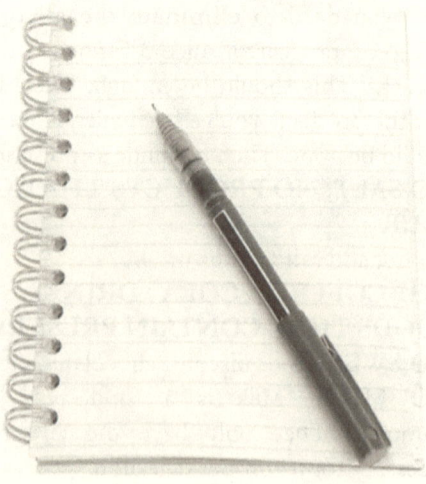

SHOPPING LIST

The very first part of the Recovery Program is to learn how to choose the right foods.

Everything you need you will find in your **local supermarket** and **health shop**, but bear in mind, there you will find **products which are not suitable for you.**

The market today offers countless numbers of food products, but not all of them are healthy options.

- Most of them are treated with preservatives (marked by name, or coded E with 3 digital numbers—ex. E 249)
- Many contain salt and sugar.
- A lot of them are cooked.

Please, first **Read the label**

Make a list of all the products you find in the shops, which contain **no preservatives, no salt and no refined sugar.**

DAILY REGIMEN

As this is a Step-By-Step Guide, we will take one step at time. Each week we will **add** new tasks, keeping the old ones.

[Full details are in the Guidance below].

Week 1

During the first week you are going to complete 1 task: Eat a breakfast of bran (If allergic to Wheat, use Oat or Rice bran). Read the Guidance for details.

Here is your shopping list:

Instead of your usual breakfast you are going to have a breakfast from the following products: Wheat bran, Oat bran, Wheat germ, Lecithin, Bio Yoghurt (Read the Guidance).

Week 2

Task 1—Have a 3 day citrus detox.

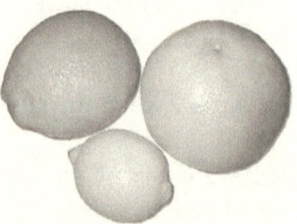

To complete it you need: 9 grapefruits, 18 oranges and 9 lemons

Note: The weekend is a good time to do the Citrus detox. During these 3 days relax at home and avoid any heavy physical work.

See details under 'Important detoxification'.

Task 2—During the second week you will begin one of the most important phases in your treatment—eliminating the fungal infection.

Until you have thrush, you cannot cure the Fibromyalgia.

Visit your doctor and ask for a prescription for **FUNGILIN** (Fluconazole) 100mg, 16 tablets. In some countries a prescription is not necessary.

Buy from a reputable company if shopping online.

The treatment continues 14 days. (See under Guidance).

STRICTLY, DO NOT EAT OR DRINK ANYTHING FOR 60 MINUTES AFTER TAKING THE TABLET.

Week 3

Add supplements and herbs. Raw fruits and vegetables are the best source for vitamins and minerals as nature has given them in perfect balance for food.

Here is your shopping list:

- Cod Liver Oil (preferably) or Fish Oil
- Sea Kelp/ Iodine
- Vitamin C
- Vitamin E (see Guidance)
- Magnesium
- Herb 'Colt's-foot' (*Tussilago farfara*)
- Herb 'Field Horsetail' (*equisetum arvense*)
- Herb Cammomile (*Matricaria Recutita*)
- Herb Agrimony (*Agrimonia eupatorium*)
- Raw nuts by your choice: Almonds, Brazils, Chestnuts,
- Hazelnuts etc. Sunflower/pumpkin seeds etc.—only raw.
- Fruits—Only raw, not dried, not tinned. The market offers a wide variety of fruits. Most beneficial for

Fibromyalgia are: Grapefruits, Oranges, Lemons and Apples.
- Carrots for juice (you need a Juicer) *Note the difference between a juicer and a blender. A blender is not suitable for raw carrots.
- Olive oil and lemon juice. Read the Guidance for details.

Week 4

Add a healthy lunch and an evening meal.

Here is your shopping list:

1. **For raw salad**: 10 different vegetables of your choice—Tomatoes, Peppers, Cucumber, Onion, Spring onion, Lettuce, Cauliflower, Parsnips, Parsley, Broccoli, Garlic, Celery etc, + Olives, Feta cheese, Oil, Red wine vinegar.
2. **For lunch**—Carbohydrates: potatoes, rice, beans, lentils, bread, spaghetti etc. (use only one product at time). When using cooked products, fewer ingredients will ease digestion.
3. **For the evening**—Proteins: Fish (all kinds of fish are good for you), Shellfish (absolutely fresh or frozen) or Eggs (Free-range if possible). Read the Guidance for details.

Week 5

Exercise at least 3 hours a day. Read the Guidance for details.

From Week 6 your daily routines are as follows;

DO NOT SKIP THE STEPS.

FOLLOW THIS SUCCESSION:

MORNING (M)

M1. PULSE—take it once a week [norm 60-70]. Write it down. BLOOD PRESSURE—once a week [norm 120/80]. Record it.

M2. ANTIFUNGAL PILL [e.g. FUNGILIN, FLUCONAZOLE—14 days]. **STRICTLY**, DO NOT EAT OR DRINK ANYTHING FOR 60 MINUTES AFTER TAKING THE TABLET.

BICARBONATE OF SODA

For 6 days take twice—morning and evening, on an empty stomach, a glass of water with 1 teaspoon of Bicarbonate of soda. Stir well and drink. Allow 30 minutes to work.

After 6 days, take Bicarbonate of soda only once a day.

Bicarbonate of soda will keep the Fungus (Candida Albicanis) away. Fungi cannot live in an alkalised environment. Candida is one of the main triggers of Fibromyalgia.

Bicarbonate of soda contributes for a normal pH, for a BALANCED HOMEOSTASIS. This is what we aim to achieve.

M3. LAZY GYMNASTICS

Breakfast:

M4. CARROTS; wait 30 minutes, let the juice work.

M5. LEMON JUICE & OLIVE OIL; STRICTLY DO NOT EAT OR DRINK DURING FOLLOWING 30 MINUTES.

M6. WHEAT BRAN + OAT BRAN + WHEAT GERM + LECITHIN + YOGHURT. Herb tea with supplements (M7 to M11). **No need to wait**.

M7. TEA—Colts Foot *Tussilago farfara*. l;lDrink for 2 months.

M8. COD-LIVER OIL

M9. SEA KELP tablet

M10. L-TYROSINE

M11. VITAMIN C

M12. MAGNESIUM

M13. GARLIC

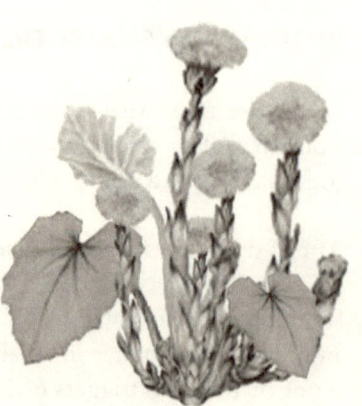

M14. SUNFLOWER SEEDS, NUTS

M15. NO SALT, COFFEE, CARBONATED DRINKS, TEA, FOODS WITH PRESERVATIVES, AND NO MILK.

Between morning and lunchtime

M16. FRUITS AT ANY TIME, CITRUSES (mainly GRAPEFRUITS) AND APPLES

M17. SPORTS ACTIVITY

LUNCHTIME (L)

L1. LAZY GYMNASTICS

L2. TEA—AGRIMONY; 30 minutes before lunch. Drink the herb tea for 3 months. Have a pause for 15 days then resume for 3 months. This should be enough.

L3. LUNCH: SALAD **80 %** + CARBOHYDRATES **20 %**

L4. TEA—FIELD HORSETAIL *equisetum arvense*. The following supplements (L5 & L6) can be drunk with the herb tea (L4), no necessary waiting time.

L5. VITAMIN C

L6. GARLIC

L7. NO SALT, COFFEE, CARBONATED DRINKS, TEA, FOOD THAT CONTAINS PRESERVATIVES, NO MILK.

Between lunchtime and evening

L8. FRUITS AT ANY TIME: CITRUSES (mainly GRAPEFRUITS) AND APPLES.

L9. SPORTS ACTIVITY

EVENING (E)

E1. LAZY GYMNASTICS

E2. TEA—AGRIMONY; 30 minutes before the meal. Take the herb tea for 3 months, pause for 15 days and then again 3 months tea.

E3. EVENING MEAL: SALAD **80 %** + PROTEINS **20 %**

E4. TEA—CAMMOMILE

E5. VITAMIN C

E6. MAGNESIUM

E7. VITAMIN E (see GUIDANCE)

E8. NO SALT, COFFEE, CARBONATED DRINKS, TEA, FOOD THAT CONTAINS PRESERVATIVES. NO MILK.

Before bedtime

E9. TAKE A BATH. Stay at least 40 minutes in the warm water. USE A BODY SCRUB MITTEN

IMPORTANT DETOXIFICATION

CITRUS DETOX During the first week of the Recovery Program you will do a 3 day detox using citrus fruits.

Shopping list:

Each day you are to eat 3 Grapefruit, 6 Oranges, 3 Lemons (this is what you need for one day). Multiply by 3—for 3 days. So, you need 9 grapefruits, 18 Oranges and 9 lemons.

How to conduct the detoxification?

—For three days you are to eat nothing else, only these fruits!

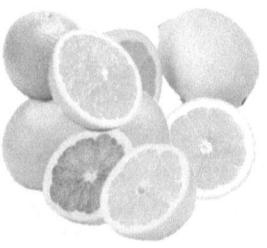

Start at suitable time for you. For example; Start at 10am and every hour eat fruits according to the following schedule:

- 10am—1 grapefruit
- 11am—2 oranges
- 12am—1 lemon; Pour freshly squeezed juice from 1 lemon into a glass, add water and drink.
- 1pm—1 grapefruit
- 2pm—2 oranges
- 3pm—1 lemon; Squeeze the juice from 1 lemon, add water and drink.
- 4pm—1 grapefruit
- 5pm—2 oranges
- 6pm—1 lemon; Squeeze the juice from 1 lemon add water and drink.

Rinse your mouth with water after every intake to protect your teeth. Use a straw for the lemon juice.

It is recommended to finish the fruit intake at about 6pm, the latest is 8pm. There is a large amount of sugar in the fruits, which is energy, and this may disturb your night sleep. During these days you will feel alert and full of energy. (And so afterwards.)

This is all for the day. Do not eat or drink anything else. If you feel really hungry, you could take one slice of wholemeal toasted bread <u>or</u> bran with citrus juice.

Complete the 3 day detoxification.

Repeat the above once a month, or at any time you need (have pain and stiffness). There is no risk for harm from this treatment, only great benefits which you will notice immediately.

The Citrus Detox combined with a bath every day is the quickest way to reduce your pain and stiffness.

Note: If you are diabetic, you can replace the oranges with lemons and grapefruits (non sweet).

If you have Diabetes, consult with your Doctor!

GUIDANCE

MORNING

M1. Take your pulse/blood pressure:

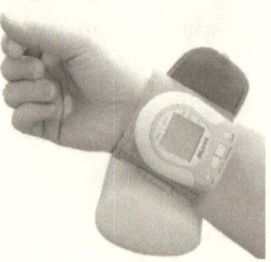

Measure once a week, at the same time. The norm is: pulse 60/70, blood pressure 120/80.

To get your measurements towards the norm can take several years.

With FM, the blood pressure is low, except in the advanced form.

M2. Anti fungal treatment:

I would like to stress on this: **If you have and until you have fungal infection, you cannot cure the Fibromyalgia.**

Do you need an anti fungal treatment? You could take a medical test of course, but there is a simple way to check it up. Take a mirror and put out your tongue. Look for a white coating on it. The normal colour of the tongue is pink. If your tongue is white coated, you most likely have a Candida infection/Thrush, which is a fungal infection and therefore you need an Anti fungal pill—Fungilin/Fluconazole (1 x 100mg tablet by mouth each day for 2 weeks).

Don't eat or drink anything for 1 hour after taking the tablet.

Grapefruits and oil from grapefruit seeds, raw garlic on empty stomach and oregano tea etc have also antifungal properties, but this way works very slowly. **Until any thrush infection is removed, the FM recovery goes really slowly.**

A huge part of the Recovery Program aims to improve the immune system, which gradually will deal with the fungi. But here we want quick recovery, so, my recommendation is—take Fluconazole tablets and after 2 weeks your health improvement will speed up.

!!! Check up your partners tongue for fungal infection as this is easily transmitted. Both of you have to take an antifungal treatment to ensure you are not going to develop it again.

Note: Your partner may have Candida but as yet no symptoms of illness at present.

Fibromyalgia is a female condition. 90% of sufferers are women. One of the main triggers for FM is Candida infection. Candida affects people in different ways. Women usually develop Fibromyalgia, while men develop Irritable Bowel Syndrome. Remember as well, everybody has his or her own weak points.

Anti fungal medicine: To obtain this you may need a prescription from your Doctor. The most frequent fungal infection is caused by *Candida Albicanis*. Symptoms of the latter are; white coating on the tongue, swelling of the intestines, vaginal inflammation etc. The fungal spores are dispersed through the blood to the whole body, the brain, kidneys, heart, bowel, and bladder. For instance, when the natural mucous lining of the intestine gets a fungal coating, this prevents the assimilation of nutritional substances.

Fungilin is a powerful synthetic anti fungal drug, which suppresses growth and reproduction of the fungus cells. Fungilin interferes with the fungal cells. The Fungilin pill is not absorbed by the body but is passed in your waste—80% by the kidney, unchanged; and 11% undergoes metabolic changes. Resistance to Fungilin is very rare.

When taking Fungilin you must ensure that you follow the manufacturer's instructions, particularly if you are taking other drugs and medicines at the same time.

Note: Here we are talking about Fungilin-**Pills/Tablets**, but NOT Injections. Do not take injections! They are not suitable for Fibromyalgia.

M3. "Lazy gymnastics"

Exercise for the capillaries and the muscles of the heart.

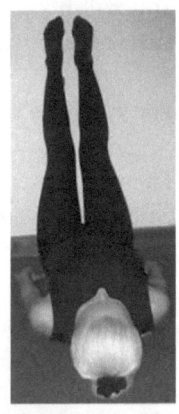

▶ at least 6 times a day.

Method of implementation:

1) Lie on your back.
2) Raise your legs vertically.
3) Shake your legs for 1or 2 minutes.
4) Lower your legs to a horizontal position.

Repeat the exercise, this time raise and shake your **arms** and **hands**.

You will feel how the blood from your limbs flows to the body torso. Your pulse accelerates to move the blood and your "always cold" feet and palms are warmed by new blood flowing to them. This is also a perfect and easy exercise for the heart muscle.

Breakfast

M4. Carrots. Eat raw carrots every day.

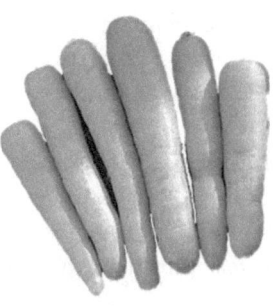

Drink freshly squeezed carrot juice from 1 kilogram (2.2 Pounds) of carrots a day. One kilo of carrots produces about 2 and a half cups of juice.

You will need an electrical "fruit **juicer**". Do not make the mistake of buying a blender; it is not suitable for raw carrots.

You can juice up to 3-4 kilos (8 pounds) of carrots a day.

The healthier option is to eat the carrots, but it takes a long time to chew them. The carrots can also be grated.

▶ Do not replace the freshly squeezed carrot juice with juice from the shop. Bottled juice doesn't work for fibromyalgia recovery.

M5. Mix 1 tablespoon of freshly squeezed lemon juice + 1 tablespoon olive oil. Stir and drink.

STRICTLY DO NOT EAT OR DRINK ANYTHING FOR THE NEXT 30 MINUTES.

▶ Apply for 3 months, then take a break of 15 days and again apply for 3 months and so on.

Why do you need to do this? The details are in "Fibromyalgia Secrets Revealed". As I said at the beginning, "Fibromyalgia Recovery Program" is about the treatment only.

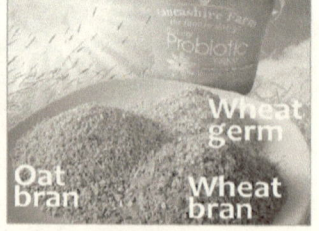

M6. Mix 3 tablespoons **wheat bran** + 3 tablespoons **oat bran** + 3 tablespoons **wheat germ**. Add natural/life/bio **yoghurt**. Scatter 1 teaspoon **lecithin** granules over this cereal. Stir the mixture and eat.

Note: If you have a **milk allergy**, replace the yoghurt with fresh squeezed orange (grapefruit) juice, but only if you get a heavy feeling/bloating in the stomach after eating natural yoghurt.

Usually natural yoghurt is easy digested (cultures like *lactobacillus acidophilus* and *bifidobacterium longum* are natural inhabitant of human intestines).

I recommend it because the good bacterium in it competes with the harmful bacteria living in the intestines.

Lecithin granules are available at any Health Food shop (Lecithin is an important building block for cell membranes. It protects cells from oxidization and is a fat emulsifier).

NOTE: Wheat products contain gluten. If you are **allergic to gluten** (Celiac Disease), replace the wheat bran and wheat germ with rice bran.

M7. Colt's foot tea *tussilago farfara*

Boil the leaves of this herb (1 tablespoon) for 2 to3 minutes in 250ml water. After 15 minutes strain and drink. Colts foot tea liquefies the excess mucous in the intestines and the lungs, which improves the body's absorption of nutrients.

M8. Vitamin D

A) **Cod liver oil** capsules; these contain vitamin D.

Vitamin D is one of the keys for Fibromyalgia recovery.

The necessary daily supplement of vitamin D is 10 micrograms (400IU) for adults and 5 micrograms (200IU) for teenagers (read the label).

Do not surpass the daily dosage. The dosage can be reduced to 5mg a day when you have achieved a stable therapeutic effect (usually after 12 months to 5 years). Fibromyalgia sufferers need to take vitamin D for the rest of their life.

Vitamin D is taken in the morning and never together with vitamin E (as it neutralizes vitamin E). Vitamin D is contained in fish roe, fish, and sea products.

B) Sunbathe for at least 14 days a year but take care that your skin does not burn at any time. How long should you expose your body to the sun daily?—Some types of skin burn easily, especially fair skin. Start with short exposure and gradually increase the time. If very sensitive, use a sun barrier cream during the first 3-5 days. Keep a bronze tan but note that vitamin D synthesis stops when the skin becomes too dark. During your summer holiday at the sea, spend more time into the water (swim, play ball games, snorkel). Your skin will get a sun tan, but will not burn as the water cool the skin.

Visit a solarium if you cannot expose your whole body to natural sunlight.

If your skin has a **natural dark pigment**, you definitely need to take vitamin D supplements and to eat plenty of sea products.

= =

An alternative to a '2 weeks summer holyday at the sea' is taking capsules of Vitamin D—5000 IU per day.

Quick calculation: A full body exposure to the natural sun light results in synthesis of 20 000 IU of Vitamin D per day. Multiply 20 000 IU by 15 days = 300 000 IU of Vitamin D. Divide it on 365 days (a year) = 822 IU. 1 IU = 0,025 micrograms vitamin D. Multiply 822 by 0,025 = 20 micrograms. If you spend your summer holyday at the sea your body would naturally synthesises vitamin D which will provide you with 20 micrograms per day throughout the year.

To be on the safe side with the supplement, please, check your Vitamin D level before taking 5000 IU of vitamin D. This web site www.vitamindproject.co.uk provides a home test kit for Vitamin D.

M9. Sea Kelp

Sea Kelp supplies the body with Iodine, which is essential for the Thyroid gland function. The Thyroid gland maintains the metabolism in the body; balance hormones, stabilize cholesterol, maintain weight control, keep menstrual cycles regular, stimulate intestinal function (constipation), provide energy (FM and fatigue), and even helps you keep a positive mental attitude (depression).

Self-Test for Iodine deficiency—How to do it?

Get Tincture of Iodine at the drugstore. At home dip a cotton ball into the tincture and paint a 2-3 inches circle of iodine on your soft skin (inner part of your arm or thigh). If the yellowish stain remains for more than 4 hours, the Iodine in your body is sufficient and you do not need to take Iodine supplements. If the yellowish stain disappears in less than 1 hour, this means your body is lacking Iodine and has soaked it up.

How to supply the body with Iodine? You can choose one of the following ways:

-**For** the next 5-10 days every evening **paint a 3 by 3 inches patch of Tincture of Iodine on your skin** and observe the time of disappearance. When you 'pass' the test, you can take 1 tablet of Sea kelp a day to ensure enough Iodine in your body.

-**Or** you can take Sea Kelp tablets; take them with water or herbal tea as follows:

   3 tablets x 30mg; morning;
   2 tablets x 30 mg; lunch time;
   1 tablet x 30 mg; evening

After 2 months take only 1 tablet 30 mg; morning.

-**Natural** sources of Iodine—add sea vegetables to your diet. Just one teaspoon of sea vegetables a day can help you regain normal iodine levels. Incorporating seafood and fish into your diet can also help. Other foods that contain iodine are eggs and dairy products—cheese and yogurt, onions, radishes, and watercress. Some foods, called goitrogens, should be omitted for awhile as they hinder iodine utilization. These included kale, cabbage, peanuts, soy flour, Brussels sprouts, cauliflower, broccoli, kohlrabi and turnips.

M10. L-Tyrosine—take 1 capsule of 500 mg in the morning 30 minutes before the bran breakfast.

L-Tyrosine is an amino acid that can be found in foods that contain proteins—meats, fish, dairy products, wheat, oats etc. It is needed for person that suffers from fatigue, depression, concentration and memory problems. L-Tyrosine is a natural appetite suppressor.

Tyrosine is precursor of the hormones threonine, a thyroid hormone essential for body's metabolism. Tyrosine gets converted in the skin into melanin, which protect your skin from the sun's harmful rays. L-Tyrosine is essential for creating adrenalin and dopamine. Adrenaline helps to fight the fatigue. Dopamine's function is to alleviate pain and control stress. L-Tyrosine has antioxidant effect that prevents cancer, heart disease and aging.

Do not take L-Tyrosine if you have high blood pressure, restlessness, heart palpitation, arritmia, and melanoma.

Take L-Tyrosine only in the morning and lunch time. Take it 30 min before meals.

Do not take L-Tyrosine in the evening. This would cause restlessness, sleeplessness and insomnia.

Do not increase recommended dose. Healthy person may take up to 7g a day, sportsmen can take up to 12g per day, but fibromyalgia sufferers should not take more than 1000mg a day divided in 2 intakes x 500mg. This amount works perfectly for fibromyalgia and also takes in account all the features related to FM and especially the condition of capillaries.

L-Tyrosine is MUST take but in recommended dose.

M11. Vitamin C 1000mg

Daily dose—3000mg to 4000mg a day divided in equal intervals (if you smoke tobacco you may need a higher dose of vitamin C at the beginning)

The market offers different forms of vitamin C. The best one is 'Timed release' vitamin C, 1000mg. It is available in different varieties—6h, 8h, or 12 hours for complete dissolving of the tablet. Ask the pharmacist and take the tablets to supply your body with vitamin C 24 hours a day.

Example:

- Time for dissolving **6h**—take 1 tablet every 6 hours, all together, **4 tablets a day;**
- Time for dissolving **8h**—take **3 tablets a day;**
- Time for dissolving **12h**—take **2 tablets a day**.

Vitamin C is not produced by the human body. The human body does not have the ability to store it. This is why it needs to be taken at regular intervals, every day. Any excess is eliminated quickly through the kidneys, so do not take all the tablets at once. Take them at regular intervals.

Natural Vitamin C is contained in raw fruits and vegetables (lemons are one of the best sourses). Vitamin C is destroyed at high temperatures. When you cook your food, you destroy vitamin C.

►Timed release vitamin C does not interfere with your teeth but quickly dissolvable vitamin C could dissolve the calcium in the teeth. In case you prefer to use quickly dissolvable vitamin C in a glass of water, or drink freshly squeezed lemon juice with water, you can protect your teeth in 2 ways:

1) use a straw or 2) rinse your mouth afterwards with fresh water.

M12. Magnesium

300mg is your daily dose. Some manufacturers produce tablets with 600mg or more magnesium. There is no harm to take more than 300mg, but it is not necessary.

Green vegetables, such as cucumbers, lettuce, spinach, broccoli etc. and fruits (kiwi etc.) contain magnesium. The plants own chlorophyll (generally indicated by green coloring) means that it is a source of magnesium.

M13. Garlic

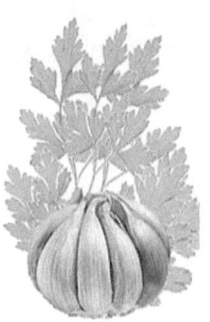

Daily dose: 2 capsules (or 1 clove), 3 times a day. If your lifestyle allows, natural raw garlic is best. You can crush it and add to your salad. (see Recipes)

Note: chewing Parsley neutralizes completely the smell of garlic on your breath.

M14. Unbaked, raw sunflower seeds, raw nuts (walnuts, almonds etc.).

Daily dose: at least 100g each day. There is no limit to the amount as they are raw.

M15. Do not eat table salt!

Completely exclude salt from your food for 6 months. **Note**: When purchasing processed shelf products in your grocery, make sure of the salt concentration on the label, and buy only products without salt. Salt irritates the tissues and results in increasing FM symptoms.

Do not drink coffee, cola drinks, carbonated drinks, tea or alcohol. As with meat, they stimulate secretion of stomach juices for their digestion, which destroys vitamin B1.

▶Note the symptoms of low levels of vitamin B1 in your body: muscle weakness, chronic tiredness, paresis (paralysis), low blood pressure, depression, swelling (tumefaction), inflamed and degenerative processes of the peripheral neural system, psoriasis etc.

Many of the symptoms of hypo-vitaminosis B1 are the same as the symptoms of FM.

It is not necessary to take vitamin B1 tablets, for it is contained in the basic nutritional products as laid out in this RECOVERY PROGRAM. But it is important not to create conditions for its destruction!

M16. Raw fruits

Raw fruits contain all the necessary nutritional substances for the health of the human body.

They contain the best source of **Glucose** (for energy).

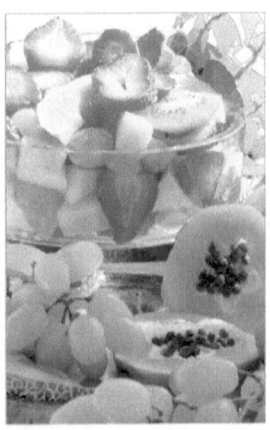

They contain **Carbohydrates**, **Cellulose** (for purifying the stomach and intestinal mucosa);

Some **Proteins** are present and plenty of **Vitamins**, **Minerals** and **Enzymes** (for the body's biochemical reactions).

If you have intolerance/allergy to some fruits, replace them with raw vegetables or other fruits for a while.

> The Bible gives good advice when it states
> ***"Every seed-bearing plant and every tree that has fruit with seed in it. They will be yours for food"***.

M17. Movement/sport activity

Between morning and lunchtime undertake some sports activity—walks, swimming, running, dancing etc. Choose the activity you enjoy, and vary it to engage many muscle groups.

A Rowing Machine is ideal for Fibromyalgia for the exercise involves all the muscles that are usually stiff. In addition, you are in a sitting position so you do not get tired. Breathe deeply during the exercises (inhale and exhale deeply).

Exercise slowly! Do not hurry!

Do not reach the point when you are tired. Tiredness leads to the synthesis of lactic acid in the muscles, which causes . . . pain. If you feel tired, stop, breathe deeply until rested and then continue.

Exercise at any time that is suitable for you, but make sure, all together, that you have exercised for 3 hours a day.

The exercises are very important for your muscles, as it is the 'food' your muscles usually lack.

LUNCHTIME (L)

L1. "Lazy gymnastics" (See **M3** above)

L2. Herb tea—Agrimony
Agrimonia eupatorium.

Drink this tea for 3 months. Take a 2 week break and drink again for a further 3 months.

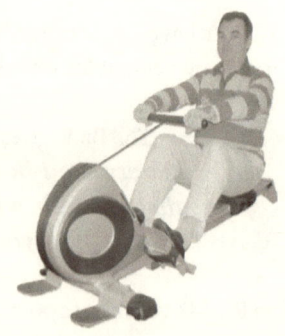

Boil 400ml water +2 table spoons of the herb for 4-5 minutes. Leave for 2 hours. Strain and divide into 2 cups. Drink each cup of tea 30 minutes before lunch and your evening meal or have a sip on an empty stomach during the day.

L3. Salad

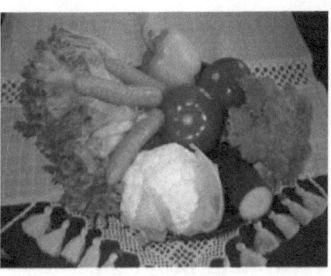

Cut 50 to 100 grams of 10 different, fresh, raw vegetables (preferably organic) of your choice, such as tomatoes, peppers, cucumbers, lettuce, onions, cauliflower, parsnips, celery, spinach etc. Add parsley sprays and 1 tablespoon of olive oil, 1 tablespoon of vinegar/fresh juice of 1 lemon, and finally 10 olives. Stir. Grate 50g feta cheese on top.

This will be your basic food for a long period of time.

Raw salads should present 80% of the total quantity of your lunch. The remaining 20% will be made up of carbohydrates of your choice such as bread, pasta, lentils, chick peas, rice, maize, potatoes, etc . . .

Do not mix carbohydrates (like bread) with animal proteins (meat) in the same meal.

Make sure that your food contains no salt or preservatives.

If you feel hungry eat sunflower seeds, nuts and raw fruits.

NOTE: "Dead" i.e. cooked food does not give but takes your energy for digestion and you feel tired. Have you ever noticed that after eating cooked food you feel tired and need a nap?

L4. Vitamin C (see above)

L5. Sea Kelp 2 tablets x 30 mg, take it with water or herbal tea

L6. L-Tyrosine 1 capsule of 500 mg

L7. Drink tea from Horsetail (Equisetum *arvense*, Equisetaceae, Bottle brush).

Boil 1 tablespoon of trimmed Horsetail sprigs for 5 minutes in 250ml water. After it has cooled down, filter and drink.

This herb is the second important component of the Treatment program.

Horsetail is a rich source of silicon that helps improve the strength of the connective tissues and dissolves metabolic deposits around the joints.

▶ To save time you can mix the herbs Horsetail, Colts foot and Agrimony together. Make a tea and drink it during the day on an empty stomach.

Only Chamomile tea needs to be made separate, so to drink it within 1 hour (see below).

L8. Garlic (see above)

L9. Absolutely none of the following:

Salt, coffee, cola drinks, tea, alcohol, refined sugar. Make sure the products you buy do not contain preservatives.

L10. Sporting activities

Exercise for at least 3 hours a day, 3 to 4 times a week.

Improve your sport conditioning gradually. Keep a soft tempo, for as long as you can.

Do not overwork, but do not forget that the general "alimentary substances" for the muscles are movement, movement and movement again. The lack of movement during the night leads to the well known morning stiffness. You are numb and movement is painful.

The type of activity is your choice and will depend on your condition at the moment. You may choose gymnastics on a soft mattress (bed), walking outside, exercises in the fitness club, dancing, swimming etc.

▶ The **rowing machine** (in the fitness club or at home) is especially suitable because it **engages all the joints and muscles**, you can control the tempo and it is performed in the sitting position.

Exercises are time-consuming. You can break them into small parts during the day. Make notes: (For example: 10 minutes + 5 minutes + 30 + 10+ and so on) but be sure you have at least 12 hours a week. The more the better.

- Walk to the shop instead of using the car. Account this as exercise.
- Do some gardening—account this as exercise.
- While in the bath, do exercises.
- Watching TV?—sit on the rowing machine.

Use every opportunity to exercise.

Repeat the "Lazy gymnastics" as often as possible. It is good for the capillaries and the heart muscle.

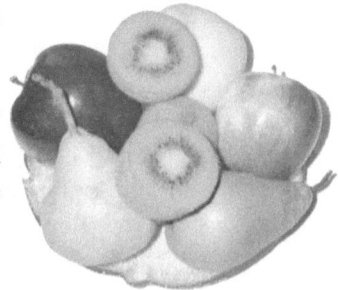

Between lunchtime and the evening

L11. Fresh fruits (see above)

EVENING (E)

E1. "Lazy gymnastics" for capillaries and heart (see above)

E2. 80 % salad (see above) **+ 20 % proteins**

Use mainly fish/sea products, sometimes chicken but preferably not red meat. You can eat eggs and Feta cheese.

Do not eat yellow cheese as its technology involves heating and also contain a lot of salt. To desalt Feta cheese, put it in a utensil with fresh water and keep it in the fridge.

NO salt or preservatives!

Deep frozen fish and meat usually contain no salt or preservatives (read the label).

Don't mix animal proteins (fish, chicken) with carbohydrates (Bread, potatoes) in the same meal.

If you are a vegetarian then do not begin to eat meat, as your body produces its own proteins more easily from vegetables and fruits anyway.

E3. Cammomile tea *(Matricaria Recutita*, German Chamomile)

Pour 250ml of hot water over 1 tablespoon Chamomile blossom, or boil for 2-3 minutes. After 15 minutes strain and drink.

Chamomile tea kept for more than 1 hour loses some of its healing properties.

Chamomile is a very strong anti inflammatory and antiseptic. It gets its anti inflammatory property from Hamazulen, which is destroyed if the tea is not used within 1 hour.

E4. Vitamin C (see above)

E4. Sea Kelp 1 tablet x 30 mg, take it with water or herbal tea;

E5. **Magnesium** (see above)

E6. Vitamin E Vitamin E: 400 to 600mg a day in the evening.

This is a multifunctional vitamin. You should be careful with it if you have **high blood pressure** (the norm is 120/80), **high cholesterol** and/or if you have **rheumatic endocarditis**. Otherwise vitamin E is irreplaceable. If you suffer from the above mentioned diseases, you will need an

INDIVIDUAL RECOVERY PROGRAM

Do not hesitate to contact me: iskra_im@yahoo.com

In the meantime, follow the GENERAL RECOVERY PROGRAM *without taking vitamin E* until your blood pressure becomes normal. This may take several months to 2-3 years. Be careful with vitamin E and check your blood pressure regularly and record it regularly.

Usually FM sufferers have low blood pressure, but I prefer to give you a warning for the 'character' of this vitamin.

If you have low blood pressure, vitamin E will increase it. Correspondingly, your blood circulation will be increased and your feet, typically always cold, will get warm; and this is not the only benefit from vitamin E.

Do not take Vitamin E at the same time as Cod Liver Oil. Take CLO in the morning and Vitamin E in the evening.

E7. Absolutely none of the following: salt, coffee, cola drinks, tea, alcohol, refined sugar. Make sure the products you buy do not contain preservatives.

Before bedtime

E8. Take a bath.

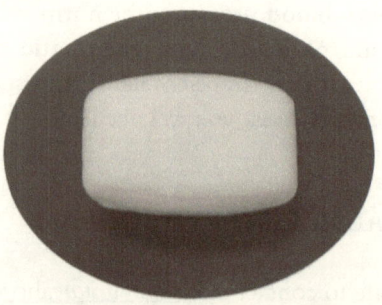

Take at least a 40 minute (up to 2-3 hours) bath every day, using a flannel mitten *, a bar of soap for the body, and shampoo for the hair.

Use a simple bar of soap (not a body shampoo or moisturizer) for your skin. Simple soap is easier to rinse off the skin.

The skin has to be left clean, free even from soap. Then the pores are open and able to eliminate the toxins.

As a result of the RECOVERY PROGRAM, the functions of the organs become activated, including the skin. Millions of sweat and oil glands begin to excrete very actively, water soluble and oil soluble toxic metabolite waste (sweat). These toxins together with the old epithelia (skin) cells should be removed from the skin every day. If you do not bathe you take the risk of itching or pimples breaking out.

HOW TO TAKE A BATH

I've received feedback from a number of patients; some people cannot bear the high temperature of the water and after 10-15 minutes they leave the bath. This is insufficient for the purposes of FM treatment.

When you have Fibromyalgia your hands and feet are usually cold and the whole body is generally cold (Low blood circulation). So, even if the water in the bath is only a little bit above body temperature, it feels too hot and you do not feel comfortable in it.

Q How to avoid this discomfort?

A Do not wait for the bath to be filled with water. Get into the bath in the beginning.

Follow this simple instruction:

Switch on the warm water (temperature to suit you); add bath salts and sit at once in the bath. At this time the water has just covered the bottom of the bathtub. The water level will rise slowly and in this way your body will gradually get used to the warm water. Soon the warm water will cover your whole body and you will feel comfortable. If the water is too hot—add cold water. After a while the water will becomes coldish—add hot water.

Stay in the warm water for 20 minutes so that the skin pores open. Then first, wash your hair with shampoo and then, wash the skin using a soaped friction flannel mitten. Do not rub the skin vigorously. Use gentle rotary frictions. Start from the forehead, do not miss ears, underarms . . . finish with your toes. Ask member of the family to wash your back.

During your stay in the bath, try to keep busy—make exercises, massage yourself or read a book . . . this will help you to stay longer in the water and gain more benefits.

Through the open pores of the skin the body releases the toxins, which relieves your muscle condition. You will notice the difference.

Before leaving the bath, stand up, wash your skin again with a soaped mitten and rinse yourself with clean water.

▶ **A common mistake:** If you don't wash your skin every day and as described above, itching or pimples may occur, then a visit to the chemist/pharmacy is made to buy creams and ointments.

Do not do this! The ointments will shut up the pores. Proper washing of the body is all that is required.

***Make your own friction flannel mitten**.

Take a piece of pure cotton flannel 25cm square (8") and fold it in half. You will get one double rectangle. Then sew 1 of the short sides and the remaining long open side together, making a flannel mitten. It will be easier and more effective to wash the body using this.

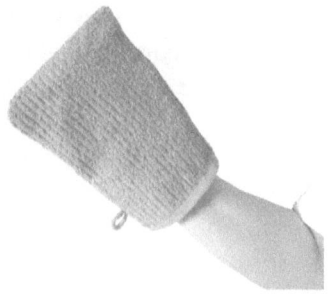

BEFORE BED

E9. **Vitamin C** (see above)

HOW LONG THE TREATMENT LASTS

COMPLETE RECOVERY

Most of your symptoms will be gone when you have done the total detoxification. (Average time to complete all detoxifications is 6 to 12 weeks, depends on your dedication.)

Would you say then that you are cured? Probably you would. Many of us associate sickness with pain, and health with the lack of it. But that is not the whole story!

From my point of view, as a health therapist, a full recovery is that stage when you challenge your body and it is able to resist. Say, you are in holiday. The restaurants do not offer your healthy food. The fresh vegetables are only for decoration, the food is salty etc. In this situation, I would say, you are completely recovered only if your symptoms do not appear again. **This is what I would like you to reach, complete recovery**. Follow this healthy lifestyle and give your body **time for repair.**

HOW LONG?

The duration of the treatment is really individual. The majority of sufferers will believe that they are cured after 2 to 6 months because the symptoms disappear. However, it is too early for such a conclusion. The disappearance of the symptoms does not mean that you are cured. It is necessary to give the body and the damaged cells **time to recover**.

Follow the Daily Routine strictly for 2 months to 2 years—Depending upon the stage of your disease (initial or advanced). Generally, the symptoms that relate to an advanced form of FM need longer time.

A TEST

When your recovery advances to the stage that you have no pain, then on some weekend when you are at home, off work, you could check up your progress. Saturdays are suitable for this. Indulge yourself with some 'forbidden' meal. If on the next day you have pain or experience any of the old symptoms, this will be a sign that your body needs more time, for complete recovery.

The most frequent diet mistakes are:

- too much salt,

- preservatives in the food or,
- mixing of too many products in one meal, or eating foods that fight within the same meal

STAYING HEALTHY

How long it takes to finally recover depends on a) how long you have suffered from FM, and b) how strictly you have followed the RECOVERY PROGRAM.

Long time sufferers will need longer time for recovery for a simple reason, their body has been in permanent Homeostatic misbalance all of this time. This means high levels of acid metabolic waste products, which unfortunately are able to seriously damage the cells. Liver and kidney cells need a long time for recovery, up to 5-7 years.

If you follow a healthy style of life you won't have pain, but every mistake will affect you.

Afterwards you will be able to return to many of your previous habits (if you wish, of course).

COD LIVER OIL

Your body will show you when to stop taking supplements and to replace them completely with raw food. Only **Vitamin D**, 5 micrograms **you have to take for life** (one capsule Cod-Liver oil).

I am going to repeat myself, but I want again to underline this:

<u>DO NOT MISS YOUR DAILY COD-LIVER OIL CAPSULE</u>

CLO keeps your capillaries open and facilitates maintaining Homeostasis. My observations show that if you miss Cod Liver Oil for 2 weeks, usually some pain appears again.

a) **Fibromyalgia comes to those w**ho by nature have limited ability to synthesize and convert vitamin D,
b) whose lifestyle limits exposure to natural sunlight (night work, northerly regions), which affects vitamin D synthesis.
c) who have insufficient fish and sea products in the diet, which affects vitamin D supply

Alcohol abuse, fungal infection and some medication side effects are triggers for Fibromyalgia.

FREQUENTLY ASKED QUESTION

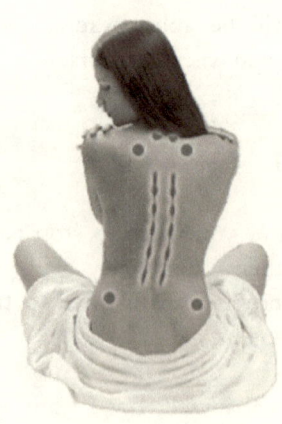

Question 1
—I don't eat breakfast in the morning. What I should do?

Answer 1
—Take your breakfast when you usually take your first meal, and carry on. Do not miss anything from your daily routines.

Q 2—I like crisps, but they are salty. Is there a substitute?
A 2—You can replace them with unsalted crisps.

Q 3—I am addicted to chocolates. Can I eat chocolates?
A 3—Chocolates are sweet and are slowly digested, which means that the sweet substance stays longer in the intestine and feeds the harmful microorganisms there. You can eat only sweet fruits which are quickly absorbed into the blood stream. But if you *do not* have a Candida infection(thrush) or Irritable bowel syndrome, if you *do not* develop gasses in the intestines after eating sweets, then that is OK. You can eat chocolates.

Q 4—My stomach is small and I can't eat all of the prescribed food. What I should do?
A 4—Reduce the amount of the portions, but do not miss any ingredient. Everything prescribed is important for your recovery.

Q 5—Can I sometimes replace the evening meal (salad + fish) with carrot juice?
A 5—Yes, you can. Carrots are a 'life' food. Carrots have a great detox power and they are at the top of the list of nutritional products.

Q 6—I am going on holiday. Can I skip the exercises?
A 6—The exercises are a very important part of the treatment but you can 'skip' them during your holiday. Be

aware, this will slow down the process of your recovery and some symptoms may return.

Q 7—You don't mention anything about drinking water. Can I drink water during the treatment?
A 7—Water is an important part of this treatment and you are going to get plenty of it in different ways—in the form of juices, fruits, vegetables and tea, of course.

You can drink water if you are thirsty, but I don't think you will be, as salt is excluded from your diet (to prevent swelling and pain).

Q 8—What I should eat when I am at work?
A8—Take your lunch in a suitable box. You may miss the dressing for your salad (oil and vinegar) as it is a bit messy, but do not miss the rest. Do not replace your healthy meal with hamburgers or other "fast food" etc.

> Keep to your diet even if you are not at home

SIDE EFFECTS

INITIAL INCREASED PAIN

From the very beginning of the treatment I have included powerful detoxification. As a result, during the first 2 to 15 days, you may experience some side effects. Your usual pain will be increased. This is to be expected and must be endured.

If it is necessary, you can take some pain killers during these few days. A good long bath, 2-3 hours, speeds the toxin elimination and rapidly reduces the pain.

This pain is not only to be expected, it is also a desired process, since it points to the fact that the healing process has started and your body has the power to fight the disease. This pain is due to the toxins present in your body.

A large amount of toxic waste will be moving out of the joints and the muscles. Toxic products cause pain, not only when they enter the body, but also when they leave it. They are being eradicated. Soon the pain will lessen.

KEEP SKIN CLEAN

The skin and the hair may become greasy at the beginning. This will continue until the oil soluble toxins are eliminated.

Take a bath everyday and use the friction flannel mitten and a bar of soap for the skin. Wash the hair with shampoo every day.

NEW STRONG HAIR

The thin and diseased hairs will fall out, and in their place, strong and healthy hair will grow back.

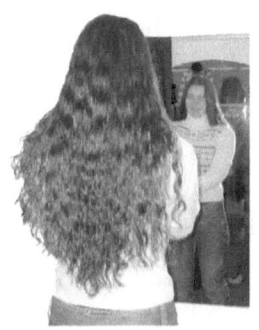

Check after 2 to 3 months and you will discover a multitude of new 1-2 cm long hairs. Very soon you will notice your hair and skin have become sleek with a healthy feeling.

Strong hair—Sleek skin—2 additional positive side effects of the program

RECIPES

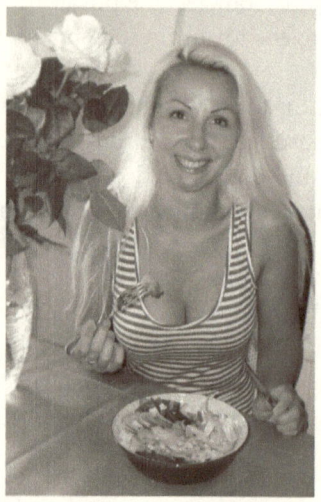

**Fewer ingredients + Simple preparation =
easy digestion and less acid waste products**

Breakfast:

1. Bran breakfast:
Mix wheat bran, oat bran and wheat germ with natural, live yoghurt.

2. Bran breakfast with fruit:
Mix bran (wheat, oat or rice bran) + bio yoghurt + segments of orange, grapefruit or other fresh fruit of your choice.

3. Scald
Bran, wheat germ and Greek Feta cheese. You could add bits of toasted bread.

Crumble the Feta cheese (and the bread), add hot water and stir. Then add wheat germ and oat bran Leave for 3-4 minutes to cool and then add wheat bran. Mix it.

4. Sesame yoghurt:
To natural bio Yoghurt add wheat bran, oat bran, wheat germ and sesame seeds (alt. Tahina—sesame paste).

Lunch/evening meal:

Salads (80%)
Salad is your main food—80% of the meal. The rest is more or less for pleasure. Start with the salad. When you finish it, your stomach will feel full and there will be very little space for cooked food (20%).

Dressings (use one of the following):

Oil + natural red wine (or apple) vinegar (not malt vinegar).
Oil + fresh squeezed lemon juice
Tomato sauce (home-made in a blender, not off the shelf)
Yoghurt
Fresh cream

Vegetables

A variety of raw vegetables guarantees sufficiency of nutrition. Wash, cut and mix the vegetables, add dressing, stir the salad.

1. Iskra salad:
Wash, cut and mix about 10 different vegetables.
These three are compulsory, Tomato, onion and cabbage (any type of cabbage is suitable—white cabbage, cauliflower, broccoli, Brussels sprouts etc).

Add lettuce, red, green, yellow peppers, cucumber, spring onion, parsnip, parsley etc according to your taste and preference. Add feta cheese and olives.
Dressing—oil and natural vinegar.

2. Tomatoes, peppers, cucumber, onion, lettuce, parsley, lemon and oil.

3. As above + feta.

4. As above + olives.

5. Lettuce, radishes, onion (leek, red or spring onion), fresh parsley, lemon and oil.

6. Yoghurt, cucumber, crashed garlic and walnuts, parsley. Crash the garlic and walnuts and add them to the yoghurt. Cut the cucumber in small cubes, add it and stir. Chop the parsley and scatter on top.

7. Spinach, cauliflower, pear, lemon, oil, garlic.

8. Spinach, mushrooms, tomatoes, carrots, spring onion (leek, red onion), dressing.

9. Cucumber, spring onion, apples, lemon, oil.

10. Celery, carrots, onion, lemon, oil.

11. Carrots, onion, red & green paprika, celery, parsley, dressing.

12. Broccoli, cauliflower, cucumber, carrots, mushrooms, green paprika, garlic, boiled egg, Feta, lemon, oil.

13. Cabbage (chopped), grated carrots, vinegar, oil.

Carbohydrate/Protein part of the meal (20 %)
The following recipes are for guidance only.

Eat simply. The **fewer ingredients** you use, the easier it is for your digestion to cope. I am not giving you the amount of the ingredients. You will adjust it by capacity of your stomach. Follow a simple rule: There is no limit to the raw ingredients. (Feta cheese and natural/bio yoghurt are raw/live foods.)

1. Jacket potatoes:
Bake a large, unpeeled potato in oven. Stick a fork in it to check if it's ready. Serve warm with unsalted butter. If you use a microwave oven, cut diagonally across the top of the potato and bake it for 10 minutes.

2. Jacket potatoes:
Serve with cubes of white, Greek Feta cheese.

3. Cooked Potatoes:
Scrub large potatoes and peel round the middle. When cooked, turn in garlic butter, scatter chopped parsley over and add pitted, black olives for each potato. Serve on a bed of rinsed green leaves: lettuce, spinach, young cabbage or broccoli sprigs (see illus).

4. Chips with yoghurt sauce
Gently fry potato chips in a little olive oil (**not** deep fat fry). Alternatively oven-bake the chips. Serve with a yoghurt sauce. (Mix 1 crushed garlic clove with yoghurt and add the chips.)

6. Potato salad:
Cut steamed potatoes, chop raw onion and parsley, crumble Feta, add vinegar, oil. Mix the ingredients.

7. Rice:
1 cup of Brown rice (or any full grain rice) + 2 cups of water. Cook for 23 minutes on the lowest gas mark/hot-plate. When ready, add unsalted butter and black pepper.

8. Toast:
Spread unsalted butter on toast (if not home-baked note salt content on label). Shake spices over (turmeric, paprika etc).

9. Garlic Toast:
Crush garlic, add to unsalted butter. Spread on toast.

10. Sandwich Pate:
Crumble Feta and chopped parsley. Mix with butter. Spread on slices of bread.

11. Garlic bread:
Crush garlic, mix with butter and chopped parsley and spread on slices of bread or warm toast.

12. Shepherds snack:
Black Mediterranean olives, red onion, a lemon (for juice) and virgin olive oil. Make a salad and eat with bread.

13. Wholemeal toast:
Homemade mayonnaise, onion and pitted olives on homemade bread.

14. Swedish toast:
Homemade mayonnaise and slices of hard-boiled egg on "Ryvita" type dry bread (try IKEA's rye crisp bread).

15. Aubergine spread
Chop and mix: baked aubergine (eggplant) + raw tomatoes, green peppers, garlic, parsley. Add vinegar and oil. Spread on toast.

16. Tuna fish:
With chopped onion and homemade mayonnaise.

17. Tuna fish:
With onion, lemon juice and virgin olive oil.

18. Baked fish:
Spread spices on top of fish fillet and bake for about 8 minutes in a microwave/oven.

19. Poached eggs:
Or fried egg (without fat, in a Teflon pan), in a sauce of yoghurt, with 1 crushed garlic clove.

20. Fried zucchini (courgette):
Easy fry slices of courgette and when ready pour on a sauce of yoghurt mixed with crushed garlic.

21. Mint Peas:
Fry 1 chopped onion until slightly brownish. Switch off the gas and add 1 cup of frozen green peas and some mint. Stir and cover with a lid for 5 minutes until peas unfreeze.

22. Scrambled eggs with Feta:
Drizzle oil into a Teflon pan, add eggs and stir until broken. Crumble in Feta cheese and heat until ready.

23. Salad "Olivie":
Dice cold, cooked potatoes, mix in green peas, grated carrots and pieces of hard-boiled eggs. 75 % veg is mixed with 25 % mayonnaise. Add lemon juice and black pepper.

24. Spaghetti:
Cook the spaghetti. Mix in unsalted butter, Feta cheese and croutons. (Croutons—Make toast and cut into small squares.

Fry until brown, reduce the heat to minimum and let them dry until crispy; add spices to taste and sprinkle on top of the spaghetti mix.)

Set your imagination free and make simple food both healthy and appealing

Enjoy!

FINAL WORDS

THE SOONER THE BETTER

I know, it is not possible from day One to change your routines, but the sooner you do it, the sooner you will feel better. Within 8 weeks you are supposed to have established your new routines.

STEADILY GETTING BETTER

Stick to the recovery program and observe your improvement. The symptoms will gradually disappear. The pain and tiredness will fade away. The feet and palms will become warm. Later on the depression will be gone.

FAMILY SUPPORT

During the process of recovery, and especially the first 2 months, family support is of vital importance. For instance family should not tempt you with 'forbidden' foods. Why not introduce your family to your healthy way of eating? This will make your task easier and your family will benefit too.

A NEW STYLE OF LIFE

My advice is, accept the Recovery Program not as a kind of treatment, but as a style of life. Keep eating raw salad; avoid preservatives and salt; exercise regularly.

By accepting the principals of a healthy lifestyle you will remain healthy and will prevent Fibromyalgia recurring.

GOOD HEALTH IS NOT A GOAL, IT IS A JOURNEY

27/06/2010
Glasgow, UK

PLEASE LIST ALL OF YOUR SYMPTOMS
BEFORE STARTING
THE FM RECOVERY PROGRAM

Name .... Date ....

....

....

....

....

....

....

....

....

....

....

....

....

....

....

.....................................if necessary, print extra page

PLEASE LIST ALL OF YOUR SYMPTOMS
After **ONE MONTH** of following
THE FM RECOVERY PROGRAM

Name .... Date ....

....
....
....
....
....
....
....
....
....
....
....
....
....
....
....
....if necessary, print extra page

PLEASE LIST ALL OF YOUR SYMPTOMS
After **TWO MONTHS** of following
THE FM RECOVERY PROGRAM

Name .... Date ....

....

....

....

....

....

....

....

....

....

....

....

....

....

....

....if necessary, print extra page

PLEASE LIST ALL OF YOUR SYMPTOMS
After **SIX MONTHS** of following
THE FM RECOVERY PROGRAM

Name ....…….. Date ………...….

....

....

....

....

....

....

....

....

....

....

....

....

....

....

...........…..........................if necessary, print extra page

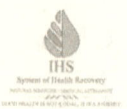

Name: _____

Date of Birth: _____

Take your Pulse and Blood pressure once a week and record the results on this chart.

PULSE & BLOOD PRESSURE
PERSONAL WEEKLY RECORD

Wk	Date	Norm 60-70 Pulse	Norm 120/80 Blood Pressure	Notes	Wk	Date	Norm 60-70 Pulse	Norm 120/80 Blood Pressure	Notes
1					27				
2					28				
3					29				
4					30				
5					31				
6					32				
7					33				
8					34				
9					35				
10					36				
11					37				
12					38				
13					39				
14					40				
15					41				
16					42				
17					43				
18					44				
19					45				
20					46				
21					47				
22					48				
23					49				
24					50				
25					51				
26					52				

NOTES

Use these pages to make notes about periods when you could not strictly follow the program, e.g. holidays, work features, family interruptions etc.

Note which part of the program you deviated from, and how this affected your recovery.

Name ………………………………….….. Date ……….…....

……………………………………………………………………

……………………………………………………………………

……………………………………………………………………

……………………………………………………………………

……………………………………………………………………

……………………………………………………………………

……………………………………………………………………

……………………………………………………………………

……………………………………………………………………

……………………………………………………………………

……………………………………………………………………

………….……………………..if necessary, print extra page

References

1. T. B. Johnston, D. V. Davies, F. Davies ed.(1958), Gray's Anatomy (37th ed.)

2. Хр. Чучков, Вл. Овчаров, Н. Стойков, Клинична Анатомия 1995

3. М. Златева, Патологична анатомия 1986

4. Т. Краев, Л. Тодоров, Ръководство по лечебен масаж

5. Проф. Д. Калицин, Проф. д-р К. Данчева, Биохимия

6. И. Крушков, И. Ламбев, Фармако-терапевтичен справочник

www.ingramcontent.com/pod-product-compliance
Lightning Source LLC
Chambersburg PA
CBHW022022170526
45157CB00003B/1317

9781450244534